MEDICARE POLICY

Karen Davis
Diane Rowland

Medicare Policy

New Directions for Health and Long-Term Care

The Johns Hopkins University Press
Baltimore and London

The Johns Hopkins University Press, 701 West 40th Street,
Baltimore, Maryland 21211
The Johns Hopkins Press Ltd, London

The paper in this book is acid-free and meets the guidelines for permanence and
durability of the Committee on Production Guidelines for Book Longevity of the
Council on Library Resources.

Library of Congress Cataloging-in-Publication Data
Davis, Karen, 1942–
  Medicare policy.

  Bibliography: p.
  Includes index.
  1. Insurance, Health—United States. 2. Medicare. 3. Medicaid. 4. Medical
care, Cost of—United States. 5. Long-term care facilities—United States. I.
Rowland, Diane. II. Title. [DNLM: 1. Health Insurance for Aged and Disabled,
Title 18. 2. Long Term Care—trends. WT   30   D262m]
HD7102.U4D279   1986   368.4′26′00973   85-45048
ISBN 0-8018-2874-0 (alk. paper)

Contents

List of Tables   ix

List of Figures   xi

Acknowledgments   xiii

Introduction: The Significance for Health Policy of Aging in   1
the United States
Directions for Reform   2
An Overview of This Book   3

1 The Health of Older People   7
Demographic Characteristics of the Elderly   7

Health Status   11
Life Expectancy and Mortality Rates   12
Self-assessments of Health   16
Disability and Chronic Conditions   16
Functional Dependence   20
Differences in Health by Income, Race, and Residence   21

Use of Health and Long-Term Care Services   22
Physicians' Services   22
Hospital Services   23
High Utilizers of Acute Care Services   27
Long-Term Care Services   27
Differences in Use of Services by Income, Race, and Residence   29

2 The Current Mix of Public and Private Financing   32
Health Care Expenditures of the Elderly   32
Sources of Financing   33
The Financial Burden of Health Care Costs on the Elderly   34

Medicare: Acute Health Care Services for the Elderly   36
Coverage Available under Medicare   38
Trends and Variations in Expenditures   39
Medicare's Accomplishments   44
Medicare's Present and Future Difficulties   46

Medicaid: Long-Term Care and Assistance for the Elderly
Poor   48
Medicaid: The Link to Medicare   50
Trends and Variations in Expenditures   51
The Eligibility of the Elderly for Medicaid   51
Medicaid Benefits for the Elderly   56
Accomplishments of Medicaid for the Elderly   60
Gaps in Coverage   61

Long-Term Care Programs   62
Public Expenditures for Long-Term Care   62
Public Programs for Long-Term Care Assistance   63
Problems in the Existing System   68
Long-Term Care Demonstrations   70

The Need for Reform   71

3 Proposals for Reforming Medicare: A Critical Review   74
Consumer Incentives   74
Restructuring Cost Sharing   75
Medicare Vouchers   77

Provider Incentives   79
Hospital Incentives   79
Physician Incentives   81

Increasing Revenues   83
Payroll Tax   83
General Tax Revenues   84
Cigarette and Alcohol Taxes   84
Medicare Premiums   84

4 Strategies for Reform of Long-Term Care   86
Consumer Incentives   87
Home Equity Conversion Options   87
Private Insurance for Long-Term Care   89
Tax Incentives for Long-Term Care   92

Reforming the Delivery System   94
Social/Health Maintenance Organizations   95

Life Care Communities 97

Block Grants through the States 100
Comprehensive Block Grants 100
Community-based Service Grants 103

Disability Allowances 104

Public Insurance 105
Comprehensive Long-Term Care Insurance 105
Expansion of Medicare 107

**5 An Integrated Approach to Reforming Financing of Acute
and Long-Term Care for the Elderly   110**

A Proposal for an Integrated Approach 110
Coverage 111
Benefits 111
Financing 111
Provider Payment 112
Delivery of Services 113

Analysis of the Proposal 113
Impact on the Elderly 114
Financing 114
Administrative Feasibility 118

Summary 118

**Appendix: The Impact of Aging on the Future Health System
in the United States   121**

References   125

Index   133

Tables

1 Average Annual Percentage Change in Age-adjusted Death Rates for Persons 65 or Older, Selected Countries   13

2 Estimated Percentage Reporting Fair or Poor Health by Age, Race, and Income, 1976–1978   22

3 Estimated Number of Physician Visits per Person Annually, Fair or Poor Health, by Age, Race, and Income, 1976–1978   30

4 Personal Health Expenditures for Persons 65 or Older by Type of Service and Source of Payment, 1981   34

5 Health Care Expenditures of Noninstitutionalized Medicare Enrollees 65 or Older by Source of Payment and Health Insurance Coverage, 1980   37

6 Medicare Enrollees, Reimbursements, and Reimbursement per Enrollee, 1967–1981   40

7 Projected Trends in Medicare Budget Outlays, 1980–1986   41

8 Medicare Expenditures by Type of Service, 1970, 1975, 1980, 1981, 1982   43

9 Medicaid Beneficiaries 65 or Older and Total and per Beneficiary Expenditures, FY 1972–1981   52

10 Medicaid Beneficiaries and Total and per Capita Expenditures by Age and Eligibility Group, FY 1981   52

11 Medicaid Coverage for the Aged under SSI by Jurisdiction, February 1982   54

12 Use of Medicaid Services by Aged Beneficiaries by Eligibility Group, FY 1981   58

13 Medicaid Beneficiaries and Expenditures by Jurisdiction, with Percentages of Expenditures for the Aged, FY 1980   59

14 Public Expenditures on Long-Term Care Services for the Elderly and Disabled by Program, FY 1980   64

15 Medicare Home Health Services, 1980   66

16 Medicare Skilled Nursing Facility Services for the Elderly, 1980   67

17 Distributional Impact of Alternative Income-related Premiums, 1985   115

18 Distributional Impact of Hospital Coinsurance on Hospitalized Elderly, 1977   116

Figures

1   Demography: Age-Sex Distribution, 1980 and 2000   8

2   Demography: Age-Sex Distribution, 1980 and 2030   9

3   Percentage Increase in Population by Age, 1980–2030   10

4   Heart Disease Death Rates for Persons 75–79, 1968–2000   14

5   Stroke Death Rates for Persons 75–79, 1968–2000   15

6   Cancer Death Rates for Persons 75–79, 1968–2000   15

7   Restricted Activity Days by Age, 1976–1977   18

8   Percentage of Population Reporting Activity Limitation Due to Chronic Conditions by Age, 1976–1977   19

9   Physician Visits by Persons 65 or Older, 1977 and 2000   24

10 Short-Stay Hospital Admission Rates for Selected Populations, 1967–1978   25

11 Hospital Patient Days by Age, 1980 and 2000   26

12 Personal Health Care Expenditures for Persons 65 or Older by Source of Payment, 1981   33

13 Percentage Distribution of Medicare Enrollees and of Reimbursements by Amounts Reimbursed, 1981   42

14 Medicaid Beneficiaries and Expenditures by Basis of Eligibility, FY 1981   49

15 Medicaid Expenditures by Type of Service for All Beneficiaries and for the Aged, FY 1981   57

Acknowledgments

This research was supported by the Commonwealth Fund. We are especially indebted to Margaret Mahoney and Thomas Moloney of the Commonwealth Fund for their encouragement and support throughout the project. We also benefited from the comments and suggestions of Lynn Etheredge, Judith Feder, and Kenneth Manton, who reviewed a draft of this report for the Commonwealth Fund. Joel Cantor, Barbara Lyons, and Carol Van Buren of the Johns Hopkins University School of Hygiene and Public Health assisted in the research contributing to the study, and Linda P. Starke edited the manuscript. We also thank Catherine Loeb and Sharon Kallenberger for their patience and perseverance in the typing of drafts and the endless process of entering revisions.

MEDICARE POLICY

INTRODUCTION

The Significance for Health Policy of Aging in the United States

During the next 50 years the U.S. population over age 65 will increase markedly. Especially rapid growth in the numbers of the very old—those over 85 years of age—is predicted. This changing demographic composition of the U.S. population has profound implications for the entire society and affects the economic, social, and cultural character of the nation.

Growth in the number of elderly people has particularly important public policy significance for the health sector. The elderly population is less healthy than younger members of society. They use more health services, and they have higher health expenditures. An increase in the number of people over 65, and especially a major increase in those who are very old, means more resources will be required to provide care for the aged. Long-term care needs of the dependent elderly, which are inadequately addressed by current programs, will grow markedly.

These expanding health and long-term care needs come at a time of economic and budgetary restraint. The United States experienced very few gains in productivity or real incomes in the 1970s. Tax cuts in the early 1980s have seriously undercut federal budgetary resources, and many state and local governments have experienced similar contractions in their tax receipts. Large and growing federal budget deficits are projected for the indefinite future. And growth in current programs financing health and long-term care services for the elderly, especially Medicare and Medicaid, is already creating serious fiscal pressures.

These trends all point to a major conflict between expanding health needs of the elderly and shrinking budgetary resources. Projected deficits in the payroll tax–financed portion of the Medicare program are generating serious concern about the future financial soundness of the program. Cutbacks in Medicare and Medicaid benefits are proposed annually. Consequently the potential for intergenerational conflict over who has the responsibility to pay for what is great.

This conflict between expanding needs and contracting resources poses both a challenge and an opportunity to design new approaches to health and long-term care for the elderly. Since those involved in formulating and establishing these policies will be affected by them, there is an incentive and a genuine prospect for long-range policies that will assure the elderly the chance to live out their years in dignity and comfort, at a cost that society can afford.

DIRECTIONS FOR REFORM

Common to most broad strategies for reforming health and long-term care services for the elderly is the need to resolve a range of basic issues.

- Who should be assisted?
- What services should be provided?
- Can the quality of the services be assured?
- How should the system be administered?
- Can the system respond to changing needs?

Beneficiaries

Should a policy apply broadly to all aged individuals, to the very old only, to those with serious functional limitations requiring assistance with daily activities, or just to individuals without adequate assets or income to maintain themselves and purchase needed assistance?

Services

Should initial steps be limited to services with which there is some experience, such as expanding home health services, or should they cover a broad range of services?

Quality

Who should have the responsibility for assuring quality? What effect do patients' bills of rights have on quality? How can families be given better information on quality of services offered by different long-term care organizations? What training of personnel is required to upgrade quality? What effect would more prominent roles, better pay, or higher status for nurses and nurses' aides have on quality standards?

Administration

Can resources be organized efficiently and incentives established to assure efficiency in the provision of services? Can mechanisms be established to assure appropriate placement of the aged and avoid unnecessary institutional care? Should organizations be given an incentive to provide quality care at the lowest possible cost? What kinds of financial arrangements guarantee stable, ongoing quality care? How should services be reimbursed? What are the relationships between reimbursement and quality, and between reimbursement and incentives created to care for certain types of elderly?

Response to Changing Needs

How can financing policy be structured to respond to changes in medical technology that improve the functional capacity of the elderly? Should the comprehensiveness of services covered take into account future demands created by demographic, economic, and social changes? What changes will be needed in reimbursement and financing as providers adjust to new incentives and as the elderly react to a wider range of choices?

AN OVERVIEW OF THIS BOOK

This book is an analysis of alternative approaches to financing health and long-term care for the elderly—an extremely important issue given the projected increases in the numbers of elderly people in the next few decades. We present a comprehensive review of currently known facts on the utilization and health status of the elderly and draw together in one place information on relevant aspects of health conditions and their implications for utilization of the health sector. The book includes new information on financial hardships from out-of-pocket health care expenditures and estimates of the distributional impact of hospital cost sharing. A projection model presents estimates of the implications of aging of the population for trends in health conditions, utilization, and expenditures over time.

Also included is an analysis of current programs financing health and long-term care for the elderly and proposals for reform. This analysis helps eliminate gaps in understanding the major financing programs and possible policy options. It stresses the importance of Medicaid to the elderly poor and notes with concern the erosion of financial protection for the elderly caused by inflation and inadequate Medicare benefits. It argues that any reform of Medicare to assure its financial solvency must also address the growing inadequacy of Medicare benefits. The book also reviews alternative innovative approaches to long-term care to fill this important gap in public policy.

Finally, a specific proposal is developed to accomplish four objectives: provide adequate financing for long-term care; improve the financial protection for the elderly for acute care services; solve the Medicare trust fund deficit; and reform Medicaid for the elderly poor. We advance this proposal in order to stimulate national debate and promote a more comprehensive reform of financing health and long-term care for the elderly with a view to achieving an adequate, effective, and stable system of financing—rather than focusing on short-term, patchwork changes in Medicare and Medicaid. While many may challenge specific features of the proposal or prefer other alternatives, we feel that putting forth such a proposal for discussion and debate will help shape thinking and move public policy action toward a system that will be better prepared for the rapid growth in the size of the elderly population in the next few decades.

Chapter 1 provides an overview of the demographic and health characteristics of the elderly both now and as projected for the future. The use of health and long-term care services by the elderly and current as well as projected expenditures for this care are also summarized.

Chapter 2 looks at the current public role with particular attention to Medicare, Medicaid, and long-term care programs. The accomplishments of current efforts and the remaining problems are highlighted.

Chapter 3 reviews the various proposals advanced in recent years to reform the financing of acute care services under Medicare. Consumer incentives, provider incentives, and options to increase revenues are discussed.

Chapter 4 examines the major alternatives for long-term care reform, ranging from private incentives to comprehensive long-term care insurance. The strengths and weaknesses of each approach are examined.

Chapter 5 proposes a major reform of current programs for financing health and long-term care for the elderly. The costs, distributional impact, benefits, and consequences of this proposal are described. The chapter concludes with policy recommendations for shaping the future course of health and long-term care for the elderly.

In order to focus on the problems generated by a rapid increase in the number of elderly, this book is limited to a review of health and long-term care needs of this sector of the population. At the same time we recognize that many of the recommendations set forth here will apply equally to the disabled and that fundamental financing reform will need to address changes for this group as well. In addition, changes for the elderly cannot be looked at in isolation from the needs of children and of other adults. Thus, where appropriate, the book touches on other financing reforms that are required to assure equitable treatment of all groups.

The focus of this work is on improving health and long-term care services for the elderly through financing reforms—rather than through organizational reforms or biomedical research, for example. This approach is taken because of the major budgetary implications of financing programs, and because the design of financing programs can have far-reaching effects on the organization and delivery of health and long-term care services. However, the book also indicates the complementary efforts that must accompany a financing reform.

We hope that *Medicare Policy: New Directions for Health and Long-Term Care* will serve to further debate on one of the most challenging public policy issues facing the United States in the years ahead. Even for those who would prefer an alternative to our proposed reform, the background on current programs and problems should be instructive. The full and informed involvement of all those affected by these policies should be sought to ensure that all relevant considerations are weighed. Out of this process should come a stronger and clearer vision of how we wish to shape the health and long-term care system for the benefit of "our future selves" (Butler 1975).

The Health of Older People

The elderly in the United States are a heterogeneous group. A few are very ill, with high medical care bills. Indeed, some of the chronically ill incur substantial medical care bills year after year. Others are healthy and vigorous and rarely use any health care services. The prevalence of disabling conditions is greater for the very old, those over 85. But even in this group, many are able to live independently with little or no assistance.

Rigid stereotypes of the elderly can lead to inappropriate policies. Flexibility to meet the needs of this heterogeneous population both now and in the future is important. Actions should be based on a clear understanding of the types of health problems of old age, their prevalence, and their distribution among the elderly population. Strategies appropriate for people with one condition may be insufficient for those with another. The complexity arises because we must consider not only the medical condition but also personal factors and social environment, as well as the interaction among these factors. Two persons suffering from the same degree of functional impairment require different levels of assistance if one lives alone and the other has a spouse who is able to aid in the activities of daily life.

DEMOGRAPHIC CHARACTERISTICS OF THE ELDERLY

In 1900 just 4 percent of the U.S. population was 65 or older. By 1980 this proportion reached 11 percent, which meant 26 million people (Census 1983). By the year 2000 the aged population will number 33 million, or 12 percent of the U.S. population. (All projections in this chapter are based on a computer-assisted planning model described in the Appendix.) As the post–World War II baby boom cohort reaches retirement, the aged population is expected to grow to 59 million, 19 percent of the population in 2030.

At the same time, if fertility rates stay at population replacement level, the younger population will not grow as fast. The age-sex pyramid shown in figure 1 will become increasingly rectangular over time as the "baby-

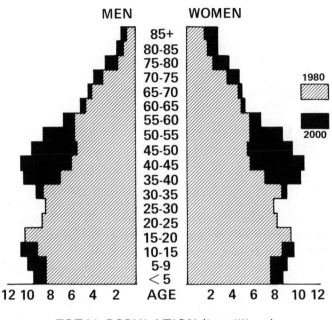

TOTAL POPULATION (in millions)
BY AGE–GROUP AND SEX

Figure 1. Demography: Age-Sex Distribution, 1980 and 2000
Source: Computer Assisted Planning Model, data file USA-1-1 (see Appendix)

boomers" age. By the year 2000 the 35–55 population will show great gains over 1980. But by 2030, as is shown in figure 2, the major increases will be in those 65 or older. The population over 64 will more than double by 2030, while the total population will increase by less than 40 percent.

This increase in the elderly population is sometimes described as the "graying of America." However, it is not solely an American trend. Most Western European countries already have higher proportions of older people than the United States does. In 1980 the elderly represented 11.3 percent of the U.S. population while in Austria, East Germany, West Germany, and Sweden they exceeded 15 percent (Soldo 1980).

In the United States, growth in the number of very old people will be especially marked. Figure 3 shows that the number of people over 84 will increase by 78 percent between 1980 and 2000, compared with 15 percent for the total population. Between 1980 and 2030 the population over 84 will triple, compared with a doubling for the total population. This growth in the very old population will have major consequences for health care utilization and spending.

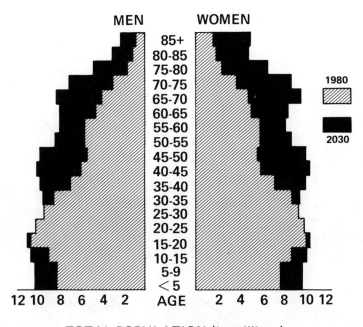

MEN   **WOMEN**

	85+	
	80-85	
	75-80	
	70-75	1980
	65-70	
	60-65	
	55-60	
	50-55	2030
	45-50	
	40-45	
	35-40	
	30-35	
	25-30	
	20-25	
	15-20	
	10-15	
	5-9	
	<5	

12 10 8 6 4 2   **AGE**   2 4 6 8 10 12

TOTAL POPULATION (in millions)
BY AGE–GROUP AND SEX

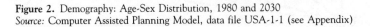

Figure 2. Demography: Age-Sex Distribution, 1980 and 2030
Source: Computer Assisted Planning Model, data file USA-1-1 (see Appendix)

The relatively greater growth in numbers of the very old will lead to their increasing predominance in the over-64 population. In 1980, 38 percent of the elderly were 85 or older. By 2000 this will have increased to 45 percent and by 2030 to 54 percent.

Among those over 84, the number of women will increase by 81 percent between 1980 and 2000 and by 206 percent between 1980 and 2030, and the number of men by 71 percent and 200 percent, respectively. The projected increase in the number of very old women suggests there will be many more women widowed and living alone. Currently 23 percent of men 65 or older are widowed or single as compared with 60 percent of women in this age group. Among women 75 or older, 76 percent are widowed or single (Census 1982). By 2000, if these percentages remain unchanged, 6.4 million women 75 or older will be widowed or single, an increase of 56 percent over 1980. People living alone or without a spouse are at greater risk of needing formal long-term care assistance.

Changes in overall family composition are also important components of an assessment of the implications of an increasingly aged population.

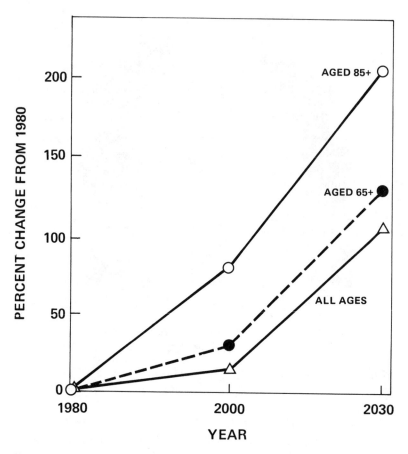

Figure 3. Percentage Increase in Population by Age, 1980–2030
Source: Computer Assisted Planning Model, data file USA-1 (see Appendix)

The marital patterns and number of children of the elderly help determine the resources available to assist with the infirmities of old age. The proportion of widowed, divorced, separated, or never married elderly living alone has been increasing in recent years—from about one-half in 1962 to approximately two-thirds in 1977 (Sangl 1983). The increase in independent living was greater for women than for men and in part reflected a decline in the number of elderly living with their children.

Pressures on the modern family will undoubtedly serve to increase the trend toward independent living by the elderly. Yet other cultural and demographic influences will make support for them less available. Simply projecting past trends may understate the degree of future dependency.

The rise in marital breakup will increase the proportion of elderly women living alone. And the reduction in average family size and increase in proportion of people choosing not to have children should further diminish the likelihood that the elderly will have children to care for them. Greater mobility has also increased the distance between the residences of parents and their offspring.

The increase in women participating in the work force means that in the future fewer elderly Americans will have a grown child or grandchild at home to care for them during the day. Nearly one-half of all women 45–64 now work outside the home (Sangl 1983), and as more and more do so, a decline in volunteer activity may also affect the extent to which private organizations are able to assist the elderly.

Yet the increased resource requirements implied by these likely changes in life expectancy and family support systems may be somewhat modified. Biomedical research can offset some of these trends if new breakthroughs provide for improved functioning in the older years. For example, an effective treatment for the painful and crippling effects of arthritis could bring relief and improved ability for independent living to the many elderly disabled by this condition.

HEALTH STATUS

There is no single generally accepted measure of health status. For the elderly, it is most easily measured by a set of loosely interrelated surrogate indicators that can be thought of as measuring different parts along a most-healthy to least-healthy continuum.

Life expectancy and mortality rates capture only the end of the spectrum. Clearly, someone who dies suddenly of a traumatic event may have had few medical needs prior to the trauma, but those who die from more protracted illness often will have used a disproportionate share of medical resources. Some conditions are not life threatening but give rise to extensive medical and long-term care needs. Several measures of morbidity are useful in detecting these needs: self-assessment of health, prevalence of specific chronic conditions, limitation of activities due to chronic conditions, and dependence on others to carry out activities of daily living.

Self-assessments of health relative to others capture general feelings of healthiness, regardless of clinical signs. This measure is a good forecaster of mortality and morbidity (Mossey and Shapiro 1982). Having chronic illnesses or being limited by such conditions is a measure sensitive to moderate levels of disability. Finally, requiring assistance with basic activities of daily living appears only in those with the greatest long-term medical needs. Each of these measures is discussed and their prevalence in the elderly population described in the following sections.

Life Expectancy and Mortality Rates

The dramatic growth in the size of the elderly population is testimony, of course, to progress in extending life expectancy that seems likely to continue. In 1960 a woman reaching 65 could expect to live until she was 81 (Census 1983). In 1980 she could expect to live until age 83, and by 2000 she can expect to reach age 86. Life expectancy for men upon reaching age 65 has increased from 78 years in 1960 to 79 in 1980 and is expected to reach 81 in 2000. White elderly females have the highest life expectancy at age 65 (a further 18.4 years). Minority women can expect to live on 17.8 additional years (DHEW 1980).

Much of the increase in life expectancy in the first half of this century was due to medical and public health advances. From 1900 to 1977, life expectancy at birth increased 48.8 percent, a gain of 24 years, while life expectancy at age 65 increased 38.9 percent, a gain of 4.4 years (Berk, Pannger, and Woolsey 1978). The decrease in risk of death from infectious disease and the substantial reductions in maternal and infant mortality lie behind these statistics. However, in recent years greater progress has been made in extending the life expectancy of the elderly. From 1965 to 1980, life expectancy for those over 64 increased 11.6 percent, while life expectancy at birth increased only 4.3 percent (Liu, Manton, and Alliston 1983).

The reduction in death rates among the aged in the United States in the last few decades, in fact, has been virtually without precedent. Three distinct periods of mortality rate decline have occurred in the last 40 years. From 1940 to 1954 mortality rates declined moderately. The age-adjusted death rates of those 65 or older decreased at average annual rates of 1.1 percent for males and 2.0 percent for females (NCHS 1982). The period 1955–67 brought stabilization in mortality rates. The age-adjusted death rate increased for men by 0.2 percent annually and decreased for women by 1.0 percent annually. Beginning in the mid-1960s, the death rates of the aged showed sharp reductions. Between 1968 and 1978 the age-adjusted mortality rate declined at a yearly rate of 1.5 percent for males and 2.3 percent for females (NCHS 1982).

Most of the decrease in mortality is attributable to the substantial declines in death from heart disease and cerebrovascular disease. From 1950 to 1975 the mortality rate for heart disease, the leading cause of death for the aged, dropped by 16 percent, and that for cerebrovascular disease by 21 percent. The decline in deaths from heart disease alone accounted

Table 1. Average Annual Percentage Change in Age-adjusted Death Rates for Persons 65 or Older, Selected Countries

	1955–67	1968–77
Males		
United States	0.2	−1.5
Canada	−0.4	−0.8
England and Wales	−0.3	−1.0
France	−1.0	−0.3
West Germany	−0.1	−1.2
Netherlands	0.1	−0.2
Sweden	−0.1	−0.1
Average, other than United States	−0.3	−0.6
Females		
United States	−1.0	−2.3
Canada	−1.6	−1.9
England and Wales	−0.9	−1.0
France	−1.8	−1.2
West Germany	−1.7	−2.1
Netherlands	−1.7	−2.3
Sweden	−1.6	−1.9
Average, other than United States	−1.6	−1.7

Source: NCHS 1982, p. 30.

for 55 percent of the overall decline in mortality rates for the aged between 1950 and 1975 (DHEW 1978).

Canada and Western European countries have also experienced declines in mortality rates for the aged over this period. These nations registered greater declines than the United States in the 1955–67 period, and then substantially smaller, but nonetheless important, declines in the 1968–77 period. As is shown in table 1, the average annual decline in the death rate of elderly men from 1968 to 1977 was 0.6 percent in Canada and selected European countries, compared with 1.5 percent in the United States. Death rates of elderly women declined 1.7 percent annually in Canada and selected European countries, compared with 2.3 percent in this country (NCHS 1982).

There is considerable dispute about what will happen to the health status of the elderly in future years. Fries argues that there is a natural biological ceiling on life span (Fries 1980). He feels that the United States is nearing this maximum and that future gains in health status will take the form of delaying the onset of chronic disease rather than extending life expectancy. Manton, on the other hand, argues that biological and historical experience does not support Fries's thesis (Manton 1982). He notes that life expectancy has been increasing the most rapidly for older women, the group that already has the longest life expectancy. If there were a fixed biological limit to life span, one might expect to see substantial moderation in improvement for those already near the limit. This has not been the case, although when U.S. life expectancies are compared to those of other countries, it appears that some of the future gains are more likely to be for men, a change that may help close the current gap between males and females in this country (Liu, Manton, and Alliston 1983).

Although this controversy is far from resolved, it seems clear that mortality rates of the aged will continue to decline and the life expectancy of older men and women will be lengthened. These changes will reflect both improved medical technology and treatment and the greater ability of many elderly to obtain needed medical care in a timely manner. Death rates from heart disease and strokes are expected to continue to decline, although at a somewhat slower rate than during the last 15 years, as figures 4 and 5 show. The mortality rate from cancer is expected to continue to rise in the absence of any major breakthrough in the prevention or treatment of its various forms, as figure 6 shows.

Predicting trends of mortality and morbidity of the elderly is complex. At advanced ages people are at risk for many diseases. And decreasing

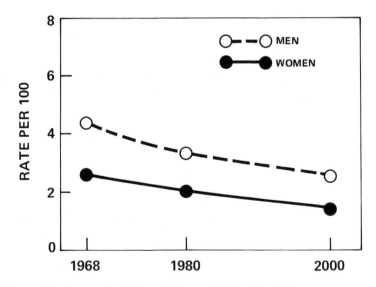

Figure 4. Heart Disease Death Rates for Persons 75–79, 1968–2000
Source: Computer Assisted Planning Model, data file USA-7-3 (see Appendix)

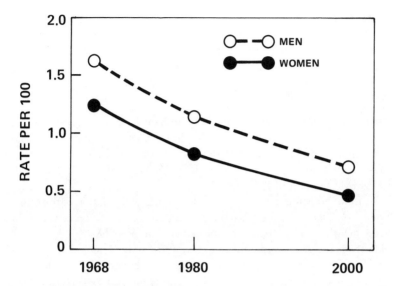

Figure 5. Stroke Death Rates for Persons 75–79, 1968–2000
Source: Computer Assisted Planning Model, data file USA-7-5 (see Appendix)

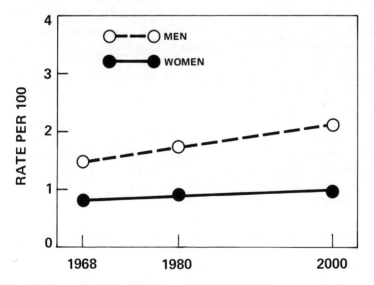

Figure 6. Cancer Death Rates for Persons 75–79, 1968–2000
Source: Computer Assisted Planning Model, data file USA-7-4 (see Appendix)

mortality or morbidity for one disease could result in an increase for another. Reductions in cardiovascular disease and strokes, for example, have resulted in an increase in cancer mortality at older ages (Liu, Manton, and Alliston 1983).

Self-assessments of Health

Perhaps one of the best measures of the health of older people is their own assessment of their status. Studies in the Canadian province of Manitoba, for example, found that self-assessment was the best predictor of subsequent mortality—even better than clinical determinations of health status (Mossey and Shapiro 1982).

In 1980, 50 percent of the noninstitutionalized population of the United States considered themselves to be in excellent health, 38 percent reported good health, and 12 percent reported fair or poor health. Among the elderly, perceived health status was more heavily weighted to the poor and fair side of the spectrum: only 28 percent thought their health status was excellent; 40 percent perceived it to be good; and 31 percent thought themselves in fair or poor health. Of this last group, nearly 10 percent rated themselves as in poor health (Kovar 1983).

After age 65 there is little variation in self-perception of health status. Kovar attributes this leveling off to the nature of the perceived health status question in household interview surveys, which asks people to report their health relative to others their own age (Kovar 1983). Another reason for this plateau is that institutionalization rates increase with age. Only those not living in institutions are included in surveys on perceived health status, yet respondents surely compare themselves to all their contemporaries, including those who are the sickest and in nursing homes.

Disability and Chronic Conditions

Another approach to the measurement of health status is determining the extent to which someone is able to function in his or her daily activities. This measure is sensitive to moderate levels of disability and medical needs. Because it is often linked to the presence of chronic conditions, it indicates who is most likely to have major medical and long-term care needs in the future.

Disability due to chronic conditions has been measured in several ways. The most common method is to ask people to report the number of their "restricted activity days"—days on which the person had some reduction in normal activities for the whole day. This would include days in which someone was unable to go to work or to school, or to carry out housework.

"Bed disability days" is a component of "restricted activity days" and measures the times when a person was confined to bed because of illness or injury. "Limitation of main activity" indicates that someone was limited in ability or unable to carry out his or her main activity. Although all these measures are based on self-assessments, the definition is somewhat more precise and less qualitative than when people are asked to rate their health as excellent, good, fair, or poor.

The extent of disability among the elderly is derived from special surveys in which older people were asked to classify their degree of disability. Several such studies have been undertaken in the U.S. population. The 1976 Health Interview Survey, conducted by the National Center for Health Statistics, found 57 percent of the population with no limitation, 5.7 percent limited in other than their major activity, 20.1 percent limited in their major activity, and 17.2 percent unable to carry out their major activity (Butler and Newacheck 1982). The 1976 Survey of Income and Education, using a similar measure, found 62 percent of the population able to work at home without any problems, while 38 percent were disabled. Earlier studies (Nagi 1972; Berg et al. 1970) reported a somewhat lower level of disability and found that 25 to 30 percent of the people reported limitation. A 1975 study in Cleveland, Ohio, by the General Accounting Office showed 41 percent of older people in good or excellent health, 53 percent mildly impaired, and 5 percent severely impaired (Liu, Manton, and Alliston 1983).

Although the definitions of disability and the degree reported vary among the studies, it is clear that many of the elderly live the remainder of their lives hampered by chronic and disabling conditions. Better indexes are needed to specify the degree of impairment and to facilitate monitoring of health status changes over time.

Disability among the aged is markedly more severe than for younger age groups. Restricted activity days occur almost three times more frequently among the elderly than among adults 17 to 44 years old. However, disability obviously does not instantly set in at age 65. It is, of course, a gradual process, with the prevalence of disabling conditions increasing uniformly with age. Figure 7 illustrates the rising rate of restriction of activity with age.

Eighty percent of the restricted activity days of the aged are related to chronic conditions, while over 80 percent of the activity restriction among the young is linked to acute conditions (Kovar 1983). Limitation of main activity increases rather sharply with age, although, as was the case with restricted activity days, there is no clear jump at age 65. As is shown in figure 8, 29 percent of those aged 55–64 residing outside institutions

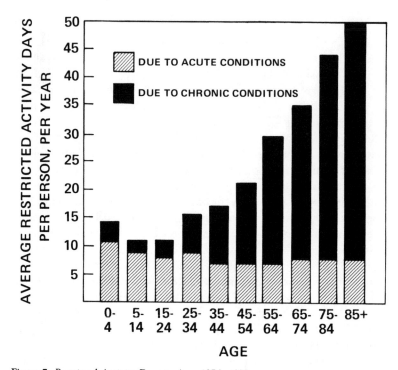

Figure 7. Restricted Activity Days by Age, 1976–1977
Source: Butler and Newacheck 1982, p. 43. Reproduced by permission of the University of Chicago Press.

report activity limitation, compared with 39 percent of those aged 65–74, 50 percent of those aged 75–84, and 63 percent of those aged 85 or older. Another reflection of increasing disability with age is placement in a nursing home. Among those aged 65–74, 1.5 percent are in nursing homes, compared with 10.3 percent of those over 75 (Kovar 1983).

The leading chronic conditions ranked by the percentage of elderly whose activity is limited by them are heart disease (8.0 percent), arthritis and chronic rheumatism (7.6 percent), senility (3.0 percent), impairments of lower extremities and hips (2.0 percent), and hypertensive disease (2.0 percent) (Butler and Newacheck 1982). Other chronic conditions among the leading ten reported as a main cause of limitation of activity among the elderly include emphysema, arteriosclerosis and other chronic disease of the circulatory system, cerebrovascular disease, impairments of the back and spine, and diabetes.

The prevalence of disabling conditions among the noninstitutionalized aged population does not appear to have changed markedly in recent years. In 1975 the elderly averaged 38.4 restricted activity days per person

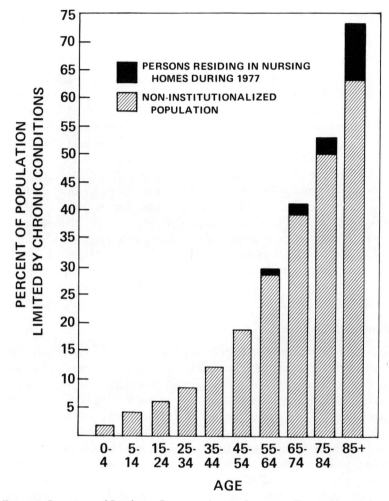

Figure 8. Percentage of Population Reporting Activity Limitation Due to Chronic Conditions by Age, 1976–1977
Source: Butler and Newacheck 1982, p. 45. Reproduced by permission of the University of Chicago Press.

per year; in 1980 this had increased slightly to 39.2 days per year. Bed disability days increased from 12.9 days to 13.8 days per person annually during this period (NCHS 1983a).

If the average prevalence of disabling conditions remains the same, growth in the aged population suggests that there will be a major increase in the number of people with chronic conditions or limited functional ability. For those not in nursing homes, the number with arthritis should increase from 11 million in 1979 to 14 million in 2000, with hypertension from 10 million to 13 million, and with hearing impairments from 7 million to 9 million.

The assumption that disability prevalence rates by age and sex cohort will stay constant over time is, however, controversial. Liu, Manton, and Alliston (1983) argue that prior attempts to estimate long-term care needs have been imprecise because of a failure to develop models to account for the dynamic interrelationship of population composition, mortality, morbidity, and disability. Both Kramer (1980) and Gruenberg (1977), for example, argue that the seriously disabled or chronically ill are now living longer because of the success of technical innovations used in disease control. They maintain, therefore, that the prevalence rate of disabling and chronic conditions will increase over time because the average duration of these conditions will be prolonged. Manton (1982), on the other hand, argues that there is no evidence that the average health status of the aged has declined in recent years, despite a very dramatic decline in aged mortality rates. Swedish studies have found some improvement in the health status of people in their seventies (Svanborg 1981).

Functional Dependence

Loss of functional independence is a special problem for the elderly, particularly for those over 84. The functionally dependent must receive some assistance. If it is extensive or if support from family or friends is not readily available in a home setting, moving to a nursing home is typically required.

Nearly all the 1.1 million aged in nursing homes have some limitation in their ability to carry out without assistance the basic activities of daily living—such as bathing, dressing, using the toilet, moving around, being continent, and eating (NCHS 1983a). Nearly everyone in nursing homes requires assistance with bathing, and at least one-half of them need help with dressing, toilet, and moving about as well.

Many of the aged outside nursing homes require similar kinds of assistance with one or more of the activities of daily living. Dependence is closely linked to age. Thirty-nine percent of those over 84 needed help in one or more activities, compared with 16 percent of those aged 75–84 and 7 percent of those aged 65–74 (Kovar 1983).

Loss of functional independence is a serious problem for older women. Since women outlive men, more older women are widowed or single, while older men tend to have a spouse to assist them. Married persons or those living with family members are far less likely to be placed in a nursing home than are people living alone. Yet support from families is not always possible. Approximately 20 percent of nursing home residents have no living relatives, and over 85 percent are widowed, unmarried, or divorced (Callahan et al. 1980). Many of the very old have outlived their children or are childless. For others, their children may themselves be experiencing health problems as they grow older. Loss of functional independence accompanied by lack of support from close family members greatly increases the health and long-term care needs of the aged.

Differences in Health by Income, Race, and Residence

As is true for the general population, the prevalence of disability and activity restriction among the elderly is greater for people with lower incomes, minorities, and rural residents (Paringer et al. 1979). Poor elderly have higher rates of disability caused by chronic conditions, although differentials by income are not as great for the aged as for other adults. Older blacks report more disability than older whites, although a much lower proportion of them than whites are in nursing homes. The rural elderly report more chronic disabilities than aged residents of urban areas (Butler and Newacheck 1982).

Poor or fair health is more common among the impoverished than among the aged with higher incomes. Over 40 percent of elderly whites below the poverty level report fair or poor health, a rate twice that of their upper-income counterparts. And a higher proportion of blacks than whites have fair or poor health. Nearly half the elderly blacks with incomes below the poverty level report fair or poor health. As is shown in table 2, even among more affluent elderly blacks, nearly one-third describe their health as fair or poor (Kleinman, Gold, and Makuc 1981).

The import of these differences in health by income and race becomes clear when another set of statistics is considered. In 1981, 3.9 million older Americans, 15.3 percent of the elderly population, had incomes below the federal poverty level. Minority elderly were more likely to live in poverty than whites: 39 percent of blacks and 26 percent of Hispanics, compared with 13 percent of whites. Of older people who live alone, 30 percent live in poverty, compared with 8 percent of those living in families. Older women without a spouse are especially disadvantaged. One-third of those living alone live in poverty (Census 1983).

Recent demographic trends will put more elderly at risk of poverty. The rising divorce rate could substantially increase the number of impoverished women. Increases in the size of the minority elderly population will also influence future long-term care needs. Today blacks represent 8.3 percent

Table 2. Estimated Percentage Reporting Fair or Poor Health by Age, Race, and Income, 1976–1978*

Race and Income	Age-adjusted†	Under 17	17–44	45–64	65 or Older
White					
Below poverty	23.5	7.2	16.9	49.5	42.2
100–150% poverty	16.5	4.6	10.7	35.9	33.3
150–200% poverty	12.6	3.2	8.2	26.6	27.4
Above 200% poverty	7.5	2.5	4.8	13.4	19.9
Black					
Below poverty	28.4	9.6	22.9	55.0	48.7
100–150% poverty	22.6	6.9	16.5	45.5	43.9
150–200% poverty	18.4	5.2	13.5	36.1	38.7
Above 200% poverty	12.8	4.7	9.2	21.1	32.8

Source: Kleinman, Gold, and Makuc 1981, p. 1015. Reproduced by permission of the J. B. Lippincott Company.

* Estimated from generalized log-linear model.
† Age-adjusted by the direct method.

of the elderly, but by the year 2000 they are expected to represent 9.3 percent. Between 1980 and 2000 the number of elderly blacks will increase by 60 percent versus 30 percent for the aged overall. If blacks continue to experience poorer health than whites, their growth as a proportion of the elderly could raise health and long-term care needs because as a group they are poorer and have aggravated health problems (Vogel and Palmer 1983).

USE OF HEALTH AND LONG-TERM CARE SERVICES

Utilization of health and long-term care services is determined by health status and the need for care and treatment, by the availability of resources, and by physical and financial access. Access to and use of these services varies by age and sex, as well as by race, income, and residence (discussed later in this section). Use of nursing home care, for example, increases sharply for those over 74; use of hospitals also increases, but less sharply. Use of ambulatory care through physicians rises only slightly with age. Elderly women are far more likely than men of the same age to be in a nursing home, and men are more likely to be in hospitals. The rate of visits to physicians is similar for men and women (Kovar 1983).

Physicians' Services

The greater health care problems of the aged are reflected in their greater use of a wide range of health care services. The elderly visit physicians on average 6.3 times annually, compared with 5.2 times per person aged

45–64 and 4.5 times per person aged 17–44. About four out of five elderly noninstitutionalized people have at least one contact with a physician during the year (Kovar 1983).

Utilization of physician services varies by health status, as would be expected. The elderly in excellent or good health and without activity limitations have fewer physician contacts during the year than those who are impaired or in poor health. Among those with poor health, one-third of those without limitations and one-half of those with limited activity have six or more physician visits annually. Only about one-fifth of those in good health and with no limited activity see a physician as often (Kovar 1982).

The elderly receive the majority of their ambulatory care in physicians' offices: 75 percent of visits, compared with 10 percent in emergency rooms and hospital outpatient departments. Telephone calls account for approximately 10 percent of the consultations, and home services and other care settings for another 5 percent. The elderly are less likely to receive care in an emergency room or outpatient department or to receive medical assistance by telephone than the nonelderly population (Kovar 1983).

There has been no change in average use of ambulatory physicians' services by the elderly over the last fifteen years, the number of physician visits per person being the same in 1980 as in 1964. However, older Americans did receive increasing amounts of in-hospital physician services over this period. Between 1971 and 1977 physicians' charges for services rendered in an inpatient hospital setting increased by 125 percent, compared with 92 percent for those rendered to ambulatory patients (Fisher 1980).

The growing number of elderly people in the future will bring with it greater demands on the health care system. It is estimated that total visits to physicians by the elderly will increase from 145 million in 1977 to 186 million in 2000, as figure 9 shows. Given the complexity of the health problems of this group, demands for specialty care should grow at an even greater rate. The expected growth in the supply of physicians, including specialists, should more than accommodate this increased demand. Nevertheless, additional training and orientation of physicians toward health problems of the elderly would be useful. Recent data show a decline in physician time per encounter for patients over age 65, despite their complex health problems, compared with patients 45–65 (Keeler et al. 1982).

Hospital Services

Elderly people are hospitalized more frequently and stay in the hospital longer than younger people. The total days of hospital care each year per aged person are more than four times those for the non-aged. Those 65

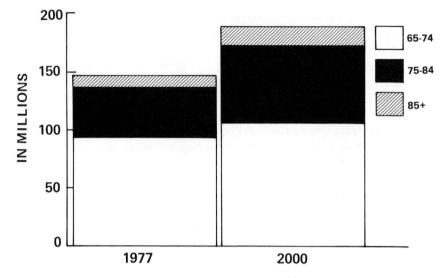

Figure 9. Physician Visits by Persons 65 or Older, 1977 and 2000
Source: Computer Assisted Planning Model, data file USA-8-1 (see Appendix)

or older average 39 hospital discharges per 100 persons annually, compared with 20 per 100 for 45–64-year-olds (Wilson 1981).

In 1980 10 million elderly were discharged from community hospitals after 105 million days of care. Over one-quarter of all the people discharged were elderly, and this group accounted for over one-third of the days. Although those 75 or older represented only 4 percent of the population in 1980, they accounted for more than one-fifth of the days spent in community hospitals (Kovar 1983).

The most common ailments for which the aged are hospitalized are: heart disease, digestive diseases, neoplasms, cerebrovascular disease, fractures (women), and hyperplasia of prostate (men) (NCHS 1983a). Accidents are a major cause of hospitalization. Serious conditions in the aged, as was indicated earlier, are more commonly chronic conditions that require ongoing medical attention, while serious conditions in the rest of the adult population are acute and episodic in nature.

From 1976 to 1980 hospital discharges per elderly person increased at an annual rate of 3.6 percent. For those over 84, hospital discharges per capita increased 4.1 percent annually. The total number of days spent in the hospital by persons over 64 increased from 60 million in 1965 to 105 million in 1980.

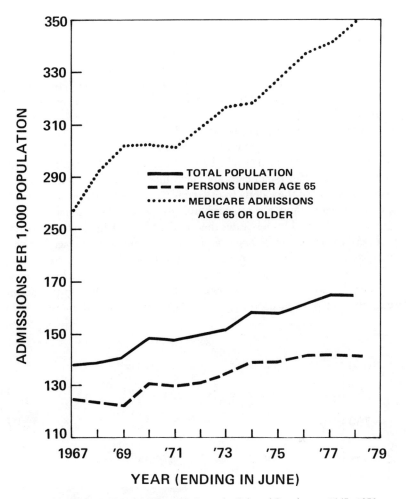

Figure 10. Short-Stay Hospital Admission Rates for Selected Populations 1967–1978
Source: Fisher 1980, p. 73.
Note: Data are for years ending in June.

The rate of hospitalizations has been growing more rapidly for the elderly than for the younger age groups, as figure 10 shows. Most of the increase is accounted for by a rise in the percentage of elderly using hospitals rather than by an increase in the number of elderly with multiple hospitalizations. From 1967 to 1979 there was a large increase in vascular and cardiac surgery and in the rate of hospitalizations of short duration. Changes in demographic structure of the aged and in insurance coverage failed to explain the difference in the rates of growth of hospitalizations by age group (Lubitz and Deacon 1982).

Studies indicate that much of the expansion of hospital utilization in the late 1960s was for subgroups in the elderly population traditionally identified as most in need of care—people with low incomes living alone, minorities, and residents of the South and of nonmetropolitan areas (Lowenstein 1971).

Certain types of surgical procedures also increased dramatically in the last 15 years. Cataract operations doubled between 1965 and 1975, and arthroplasty nearly tripled (Drake 1978). Comparison of various procedures indicates that older Americans are much more likely to undergo surgical intervention than the elderly in other countries. Coronary bypass surgery, cataract surgery, and hip replacements are performed at a substantially greater rate in the United States than in the United Kingdom or Canada.

Major increases can be expected in use of hospitals by the aged, if past patterns continue. Hospital patient days for the aged are expected to reach 273 million in 2000—almost tripling the use of hospital care by the aged in just 20 years. As figure 11 shows, the proportion of all hospital patient days accounted for by people age 65 and over is expected to increase from

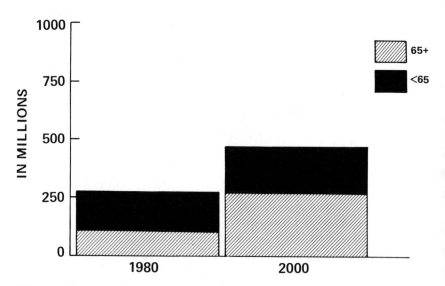

Figure 11. Hospital Patient Days by Age, 1980 and 2000
Source: Computer Assisted Planning Model, data file USA-8-6 (see Appendix)

38 percent in 1980 to 58 percent by 2000 (K. Davis 1983). Thus elderly Americans have an impact on hospital use that is disproportionate to the size of the group.

High Utilizers of Acute Care Services

Although many of the elderly are healthy and rarely use health care services, others have multiple chronic health conditions requiring extensive care and treatment. Recent studies show that 7 percent of the aged account for 65 percent of all Medicare payments for the elderly (HCFA 1983b). A study of Medicare beneficiaries in Colorado found that 18 percent of enrollees account for 80 percent of the cost of services delivered in an average year and that high utilizers in one year tended to remain high utilizers in the next (McCall and Wai 1983).

A third study of Medicare beneficiaries using hospital services found that those who were hospitalized in 1974 had a 34 percent chance of being hospitalized in 1975, while those not hospitalized in 1974 had only a 14 percent chance. The authors also found that those whose Medicare expenditures exceeded $10,000 in 1974 were 20 times as likely as other beneficiaries to have Medicare expenditures exceeding $10,000 in 1975 (Anderson and Knickman 1984).

Studies of use of services by the elderly in Canada have documented similar trends. A small proportion of the elderly account for most of the utilization. In a study in Manitoba, 9 percent accounted for 35 percent of all physician visits, and 10 percent used 78 percent of all hospital days. On the other hand, 20 percent did not visit a physician at all, and 80 percent did not use hospital services (Roos and Shapiro 1981).

Long-Term Care Services

Long-term care services include nursing home, home health, day hospital, and hospice care, and a host of health and social services to those who are functionally dependent. These services may be provided formally by hospitals, home health agencies, private duty nurses, or other organizations or individuals, or they may be provided informally by family, neighbors, volunteer organizations, or friends.

Little systematic data exist in the United States on utilization of long-term care services other than nursing homes. Growth in home health and hospice services may have received a boost with legislative changes in the early 1980s, but systematic reporting of the effect of these changes is not yet available.

As we noted earlier, nursing home placement is closely linked to age. Out of 1.3 million people in nursing homes in 1977, 1.1 million were 65 or older. The risk of nursing home placement increases very sharply with advancing age. For example, 1.5 percent of Americans aged 65–74 as compared with 22 percent of those over 84 are in nursing homes (Kovar 1983).

The increasing numbers of the elderly, especially the very old, have contributed to an increase in the absolute numbers of aged persons with serious health care problems. The number of persons 65 or older residing in nursing homes increased from fewer than 550,000 in 1964 to over 1.1 million in 1977. This represents an increase from 2.5 percent in 1963 to 4.8 percent in 1977 (NCHS 1981). This rise in institutionalization may reflect an increased frailty; it may also reflect greater financial coverage and availability of nursing home care.

The age of nursing home residents means that most suffer from the chronic multiple conditions associated with old age. Almost everyone in a nursing home has one or more impairments, with an average of four per resident. The most common chronic condition was arteriosclerosis, affecting nearly one-half of all residents. Over one-third had heart problems, and almost one-third were senile. One-quarter of all residents were impaired by rheumatism or arthritis. The prevalence of each of these conditions increases with age. Female residents had higher rates of arteriosclerosis, hypertension, and senility than males (NCHS 1981).

Studies of determinants of nursing home placement show that high levels of functional dependency are the most powerful predictor of institutionalization. Compared to an average person 65 years old or older, an individual who requires assistance using the toilet or eating is 16 times more likely to live in a nursing home (Weissert and Scanlon 1982).

Among the elderly in nursing homes, 86 percent need assistance with bathing and 69 percent with dressing; 66 percent require help walking or are bedfast; 53 percent need aid using the toilet; and 45 percent are incontinent (NCHS 1981). The proportion of residents requiring assistance increases with age.

Other important determinants of nursing home placement are: the absence of a spouse, the presence of chronic mental and physical conditions, and advanced age (over 84). Access to nursing homes, however, is limited by economic circumstances. A poor person is less likely to live in a nursing home even when other determinants of placement are controlled for. In fact, in areas where the supply of nursing home beds is short, the poor are often unable to find a nursing home willing to take them no matter how severe their disabling condition (Scanlon 1980; Weissert and Scanlon 1982).

This does not mean, however, that people in nursing homes are not poor. Nearly one-half of residents are impoverished and qualify for Medicaid assistance to pay their nursing home bills. For the most part, these people were not poor when they entered the nursing home; they became impoverished and eligible for Medicaid when the cost of care in the nursing home exhausted their personal resources.

If the same proportion of elderly in each age-sex cohort move to nursing homes in the future, the aged in these homes should increase from 1.1 million in 1977 to 1.8 million by 2000. Similar growth will occur in those functionally dependent aged requiring long-term care services in the home or community. The number of aged confined to bed is expected to increase from 460,000 in 1977 to 660,000 in 2000. Those needing help getting around within their own home will increase from 1.9 million in 1977 to 2.7 million in 2000.

These projections, based on historical experience, are not immutable. Greater efforts can be made to care for the elderly at home or on an ambulatory basis, rather than relying as heavily as in the past on inpatient hospital and nursing home care. Technological advances to prevent or better control chronic conditions may markedly reduce reliance on high-cost institutional care. But if no steps are taken, serious strains on the health care system could be generated. It is also possible that people will go without services.

Differences in Use of Services by Income, Race, and Residence

Low-income elderly, blacks, and residents of rural areas use fewer health care services relative to other groups that are commensurate with health status (Paringer et al. 1979). Since most older Americans have Medicare to help finance basic medical services, use differentials cannot be explained by lack of health insurance coverage. Some of the observed differences may reflect financial barriers attributable to the substantial cost-sharing requirements of Medicare. Lack of health care resources in poor inner-city and rural areas may also account for some of the observed differentials.

The 1977 National Medical Care Expenditure Survey, conducted by the Department of Health and Human Services, revealed notable differences in utilization between whites and minorities. Elderly blacks visited a physician on average five times a year, compared with six times per

elderly white. When adjusted for differences in health status, these differentials are even greater. Elderly blacks in fair or poor health saw a
physician less frequently than whites of comparable health. Differences
also occur in source and ease of care. Over one-half of the elderly blacks
used an emergency room or hospital outpatient department to obtain
medical care, while less than one-third of the elderly whites obtained care
from this source. Elderly whites were more likely to receive care from a
private physician. And blacks traveled further than whites to obtain care
and waited longer for it when they arrived (NCHSR 1982).

Although the poor have more health problems than the nonpoor, the
elderly poor receive less ambulatory care than elderly people at higher
income levels. Minorities are especially disadvantaged. As table 3 shows,
elderly blacks in fair or poor health with incomes below the poverty level
register 7.5 physician visits per year compared with 8 for elderly poor
whites and 12 for elderly upper-income whites in fair or poor health
(Kleinman, Gold, and Makuc 1981). Thus, even after one adjusts for
health status, the poor and minorities use fewer health services.

In Canada, where universal insurance covers most health costs for the
elderly, these differentials do not appear. There is no difference by income
in ambulatory visits of Manitoba's elderly, and those with low income are
more likely to be hospitalized than those with higher incomes (Roos and

Table 3. Estimated Number of Physician Visits per Person Annually, Fair or Poor Health,
by Age, Race, and Income, 1976–1978*

Race and Income	Age-adjusted†	Under 17	17–44	45–64	65 or Older
White					
Below poverty	9.98	9.14	10.36	10.95	8.90
100–150% poverty	10.68	11.36	10.36	10.95	9.61
150–200% poverty	11.34	13.30	10.36	10.95	10.66
Above 200% poverty	13.51	17.16	12.69	10.95	11.90
Black					
Below poverty	8.97	5.68	11.39	9.39	7.58
100–150% poverty	9.42	7.06	11.39	9.39	8.18
150–200% poverty	9.85	8.26	11.39	9.39	9.08
Above 200% poverty	10.65	10.67	11.39	9.39	10.14

Source: Kleinman, Gold, and Makuc 1981, p. 1016. Reproduced by permission of the
J. B. Lippincott Company.

* Estimated from generalized log-linear model.
† Age-adjusted by the direct method.

Shapiro 1981). It appears that when services are completely insured, almost all elderly who perceive their health as poor are in contact with the health system and that low-income elderly use services at a level commensurate with their health status.

The Current Mix of Public and Private Financing

The United States has a mixed public-private approach to the financing of health care services for its population. Most working people and their families are covered by private health insurance provided through their place of employment. For those outside the work force, such as the aged and disabled, public programs have been developed. Despite this, direct payments for health care by the aged and supplementary private health insurance coverage continue to be quite important. Thus even for older Americans, financing is a patchwork of public and private coverage, with some receiving comprehensive coverage from a combination of plans and others continuing to incur quite substantial out-of-pocket outlays.

Health Care Expenditures of the Elderly

Health care expenditures have been increasing at a particularly rapid rate in recent years. In 1982 a total of $322 billion, or 10.5 percent of the GNP, was spent in the United States in this sector (Gibson, Waldo, and Levit 1983). In just three short years, health spending increased by 50 percent—considerably faster than inflation in the economy and growth in family incomes.

The growth in expenditures has been even more rapid for the elderly. In 1977 some $43 billion were spent on health care services for the elderly, a figure representing 29 percent of all personal health care expenditures. By 1981 this had increased to $83 billion—33 percent of all personal health care spending (OFAA 1982).

The average expenditure for personal health care services for someone 65 or older in 1981 was $3,140, compared with $828 for someone under 65. Much of this difference reflects greater use of hospital and nursing home care by the aged. For example, the average annual per capita hospital expenditure of the aged was $1,381 in 1981, compared with $392 for the non-aged. For nursing homes, the average figure was $732 per elderly person, compared with $30 for the rest of the population. Differences also exist in expenditures for ambulatory care services: spending on physicians per aged person in 1981 was $589, compared with $189 for the non-aged (OFAA 1982).

With the growth in the number of old people, total health care expenditures for the aged are expected to increase from about $83 billion in 1981 to almost $200 billion in 2000, in constant 1980 dollars (K. Davis 1983). Extended life expectancy and improved health of the elderly will bring with it a cost—one that is clearly affordable to a growing and prosperous society. But developing innovative approaches to providing quality health care more economically does represent a challenge.

Sources of Financing

As we have indicated, funds for health care for the elderly come from several sources. In 1981 Medicare and Medicaid spent $49 billion on health care for the elderly (see figure 12). Medicare paid 45.3 percent ($1,422) of the per capita bill for the elderly that year. The other sources

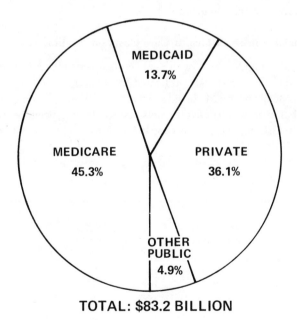

TOTAL: $83.2 BILLION

Figure 12. Personal Health Care Expenditures for Persons 65 or Older by Source of Payment, 1981
Source: HCFA, unpublished statistics, November 1982.
Note: Figures are for calendar year.

of funding were Medicaid (13.7 percent, or $430 of the per capita bill), other public programs (4.9 percent, or $154), and private payments, including private health insurance and out-of-pocket expenses (36.1 percent, or $1,132) (OFAA 1982).

The mix of public and private payment varies by type of health service. As is shown in table 4, hospital care is financed publicly to a greater extent than other services. Of the $36.6 billion spent on hospital care for the elderly in 1981, $31.3 billion (86 percent) were paid by public programs. Of that, Medicare was by far the largest, accounting for $27.1 billion (74 percent) (OFAA 1982).

In contrast, 58 percent of the $15.6 billion spent on physicians' services for the elderly was covered by public programs, nearly all of it by Medicare. And of the $19.4 billion spent on nursing home care, only 50 percent was paid publicly, nearly all of it (48 percent of the total) by Medicaid (OFAA 1982).

Most other services are paid for privately by the elderly. For example, 82 percent of the $5.1 billion spent on prescription drugs and drug sundries is paid by the consumers. Dental care in the amount of $2.4 billion is almost totally privately financed.

The Financial Burden of Health Care Costs on the Elderly

The financial burden of these health care costs is very unevenly distributed among the elderly, for, as was indicated in chapter 1, their health care needs vary. Medicare and Medicaid assist many of those with serious health problems, but even with these programs many elderly, especially the near-poor, can suffer financially from health care bills.

Table 4. Personal Health Expenditures for Persons 65 or Older by Type of Service and Source of Payment, 1981

| | Personal Health Expenditures ($ billions) | Percentage Distribution Source of Payment | | | |
		Total	Medicare	Other Public	Private
Total	$83.2	100.00	45.3	18.6	36.1
Hospital	36.6	100.00	74.0	11.5	14.5
Physician	15.6	100.00	54.5	3.2	42.3
Nursing home	19.4	100.00	2.1	48.4	49.5
Drugs	5.1	100.00	—	17.6	82.4
Dental	2.4	100.00	—	4.2	95.8
Other	4.1	100.00	40.0	12.5	47.5

Source: Unpublished statistics, Bureau of Data Management and Strategy, Division of National Cost Estimates, Baltimore, November 1982.

Because the elderly vary so much, the distribution of health expenditures for this group is very skewed. In 1980, 7 percent of the elderly spent over $5,000 on health care; 15 percent spent $1,000–$5,000; and nearly half spent less than $200 (NCHS 1983b).

Despite gains in recent years, the elderly, for the most part, are not a prosperous group. Half of the families with an elderly member had incomes below twice the poverty level in 1981, which means that their annual income in that year was less than $9,000. In contrast, 30 percent of persons in families without an aged member have incomes under twice the poverty level. In 1981, 15.3 percent of the aged had incomes below the poverty level, compared with 14 percent of all Americans (Census 1983).

Despite Medicare and Medicaid, many elderly people already face serious financial burdens in meeting their health care expenses. In 1980, 6 percent of the elderly had out-of-pocket health care expenses (not counting health insurance premiums) of more than $1,000 and 16 percent of more than $500 (Kovar 1983).

This personal spending by the elderly is expected to continue to grow. The Congressional Budget Office estimates that the out-of-pocket costs for Medicare cost sharing will be $505 per enrollee in 1984. The Supplementary Medical Insurance (the Part B of Medicare that covers physician services) premium, cost sharing, and deductible will account for 80 percent of this total. (The premium alone is now $175 per year.) In addition, it is estimated that the average beneficiary will pay a further $550 in 1984 for noninstitutional care not covered by Medicare, most notably prescription drugs and dental care. If nursing home care were included, it would add another $650 per person, for a total out-of-pocket cost to the elderly of $1,705 (CBO 1983).

The incidence of illness and the financial burden of cost sharing are not related to ability to pay. Out-of-pocket health care expenditures, excluding nursing home care, represent 2 percent of total income in families with incomes in excess of $30,000 and 21 percent of the total in families with incomes less than $5,000 (CBO 1983). Cost-sharing requirements by their very design mean that those who are ill and use services bear the burden. The chronically ill and other high utilizers of care are most likely to incur large personal liability for Medicare cost sharing and uncovered services and charges.

Medicare supplementary ("Medigap") policies are purchased by the elderly primarily to fill the gaps resulting from Medicare deductibles, coinsurance, and an occasional uncovered benefit such as private nursing. Its widespread use shows the elderly's desire for "first dollar" coverage and the difficulty of relying on patient cost sharing as a means of reducing utilization.

However, not all older Americans can afford Medigap. Overall, 66 percent of the elderly have private health insurance in addition to Medicare. Of the poor or near-poor (individuals with income below 125 percent of the poverty level), however, 47 percent have private insurance, compared with 78 percent of the high-income elderly (individuals with incomes above 400 percent of the poverty level) (Wilensky and Berk 1983). The heavy financial burden of health care on those with lower incomes is in part a reflection of their inability to afford such supplementary insurance.

The use of private health insurance to supplement Medicare increases with education as well as income. Only 42 percent of the elderly with less than 8 years of eduation had private insurance coverage, in contrast to 82 percent of those with 13 or more years of schooling. It is interesting, however, that those in excellent health are more likely to have private insurance coverage (73 percent are covered) than those in poor health (only 49 percent have private coverage) (HCFA 1983a).

Those with Medicare and private insurance coverage spend more on health care than those with just Medicare. As is shown in table 5, which consists of data from the National Medical Care Utilization and Expenditure Survey, the mean total expenditure per person with Medicare and private coverage in 1980 was $1,818, compared with $1,087 for those with only Medicare coverage. Yet the mean out-of-pocket expenditure of $364 for the former group was higher than the $318 out-of-pocket cost for the latter (HFCA 1983a). The elderly who purchase private insurance to supplement Medicare appear to pay more for health insurance coverage without a commensurate reduction in financial burden. The low-income elderly with both Medicare and Medicaid have the lowest out-of-pocket expenditures ($133), as would be expected. However, overall expenditures for this group are 3 times greater than for other elderly. This reflects the poorer health status of the low-income elderly.

MEDICARE: ACUTE HEALTH CARE SERVICES FOR THE ELDERLY

For 15 years the Medicare program has operated with relatively little controversy—steadily paying the hospital and physician bills of millions of elderly and disabled Americans. It has won widespread support by relieving the financial burden of health care bills on the elderly and their families and by ensuring financial access to hospital and physician services for many of the nation's most vulnerable and critically ill citizens.

Yet despite its noncontroversial past the program is likely to come under intense scrutiny in the years ahead. Medicare spent $47 billion in 1982,

Table 5. Health Care Expenditures of Noninstitutionalized Medicare Enrollees 65 or Older by Source of Payment and Health Insurance Coverage, 1980

		Health Insurance Coverage			
Source of Payment	Total	Medicare Only	Medicare and Medicaid Only	Medicare and Private Health Insurance Only	Medicare and Other Plans
Total expenditures ($ thousands)					
Out-of-pocket	7,637,654	1,569,841	315,670	5,698,904	53,239
Medicare	23,275,509	3,597,149	4,270,217	15,482,361	25,782
Medicaid	3,067,797	—	2,727,522	—	0
Private plans	6,059,122	—	—	—	0
Other sources	1,222,014	73,344	12,926	823,210	312,535
Unknown source/ unpaid amount	310,128	68,299	56,663	184,812	354
Total	41,672,226	5,364,437	7,437,995	28,477,883	391,911
Percentage of total expenditures					
Out-of-pocket	18.3	29.3	4.2	20.0	13.6
Medicare	56.1	67.1	57.4	54.4	6.6
Medicaid	7.4	—	36.7	—	0.0
Private plans	14.5	—	—	20.9	0.0
Other sources	2.9	1.4	.2	2.9	79.8
Unknown source/ unpaid amount	.7	1.3	.7	.7	.1
Total	100.0	100.0	100.0	100.0	
Mean expenditure per person					
Out-of-pocket	$ 328	$ 318	$ 133	$ 364	$ 184
Medicare	1,005	729	1,799	988	89
Medicaid	131	—	1,149	—	0.0
Private plans	260	—	—	380	0.0
Other sources	53	15	5	53	1,078
Unknown source/ unpaid amount	13	14	24	12	1
Total	1,791	1,087	3,133	1,818	1,352

Source: HCFA 1983a, p. 6.

up 17 percent over the previous year (OMB 1983). It is a major item in the national budget, accounting for $1 out of every $15 spent by the federal government and two-thirds of all federal health outlays. Efforts to reduce budgetary expenditures are increasingly focusing on the program. Recent legislative changes have tightened hospital payment practices under Medicare, and forecasts of future deficits in the hospital portion of the program are adding to pressures to make more fundamental changes.

Coverage Available under Medicare

The primary objective of Medicare is to protect the aged and disabled against large medical outlays. The program also seeks to eliminate financial barriers that discourage these groups from seeking medical care. Medicare covers Americans 65 or older who are entitled to receive social security or railroad retirement benefits. As a result, about 95 percent of the elderly are covered (HCFA 1983a). Beginning in July 1973, Medicare coverage was also extended to people who have been permanently and totally disabled for two years or more and to those with end-stage renal disease. In 1981 a total of 29 million aged and disabled people, representing 12.4 percent of the U.S. population, were enrolled in Medicare (HCFA 1983b).

The program provides insurance coverage for acute medical care services. It consists of two parts: Hospital Insurance (HI), known as Part A, and Supplementary Medical Insurance (SMI), Part B. The HI program primarily covers short-stay hospital care, limited post-hospital care in skilled nursing facilities, and home health services. SMI covers physician, outpatient hospital, additional home health care, and some ambulatory services. Medicare does not cover prescription or over-the-counter drugs, preventive services, dental care, routine eye examinations, eyeglasses, hearing aids, or long-term institutional services.

HI coverage is automatic for all social security and railroad retirement beneficiaries. Those covered under HI may voluntarily enroll in SMI by paying a premium. Any elderly persons ineligible for social security can purchase HI coverage under Medicare directly, at a rate currently set at $113 per month (CBO 1983).

The HI component of Medicare is financed by a payroll tax of 2.6 percent of wages. Employers and employees covered by the program each contribute 1.3 percent of earnings, up to a maximum of $35,700. The rate is scheduled to increase to 1.35 percent in 1985 and to 1.45 percent in 1986 (Rivlin 1983). Since 1966 this tax has been assessed in conjunction with the social security payroll tax, but the revenues for the Medicare portion are part of a separately administered trust fund, the Hospital Insurance Trust Fund. Current law does not permit the use of general revenues if the HI Trust Fund balance falls below the level required to pay benefits.

SMI coverage is optional and financed by general tax revenues and monthly premium contributions of the enrollees. The premium as of January 1984 was $14.60 per month, up from $3 in 1966, when the program began. The premium covers about 25 percent of the SMI costs, and the remainder is financed by general revenues. When Medicare was enacted, the premiums were intended to cover half the cost of SMI, but the share paid by the premium has declined over time as increases in program costs have outpaced premium increases.

Not everyone eligible for HI coverage elects to be covered for physician services under SMI. In 1982 fully 99 percent of the elderly covered under HI purchased SMI coverage, but only 92 percent of the disabled enrolled (CBO 1983). The poor elderly and disabled are frequently enrolled for Medicare SMI services by state Medicaid programs. Under this "buy-in" arrangement, Medicaid pays the SMI premium for Medicare beneficiaries whose incomes fall below the state's Medicaid income level.

HI covers inpatient hospital care for 90 days of any illness (a new illness is defined as beginning when a beneficiary has not been in a hospital or nursing home for 60 consecutive days), plus a 60-day lifetime reserve. The beneficiary pays a first-day deductible indexed to the cost of hospital care ($356 in 1984, up from $40 in 1966, when the program began). In addition, the beneficiary pays one-fourth of the deductible for days 61 through 90 of hospital care, and one-half of the deductible for each day of the lifetime reserve. For skilled nursing facility care, the beneficiary pays a coinsurance charge that is set at one-eighth of the hospital deductible for days 21 through 100 of care.

For physician services, the beneficiary is responsible for the first $75 of services, 20 percent of all Medicare allowable charges, and any physicians' charges beyond those allowed by Medicare. On about one-half of Medicare claims, physicians charge more than the allowable rate (Ferry et al. 1980). These cost-sharing requirements are in addition to the premiums for SMI coverage and can result in substantial out-of-pocket expenditures for many elderly people.

Trends and Variations in Expenditures

Medicare expenditures have risen rapidly throughout the last 15 years. As table 6 shows, reimbursement for services increased from $4.5 billion in 1967, the first full year of the program, to nearly $40 billion in 1981. Enrollees over this period went from 19.5 million aged to 29 million aged and disabled (HCFA 1983b).

The major increase in Medicare enrollment occurred in 1973 after the Social Security Act amendments of 1972 added coverage of the permanently and totally disabled and those with renal disease to the Medicare program. In 1981 almost 3 million Medicare enrollees were covered because of disability, including 27,000 with end-stage renal disease (HCFA 1983b).

That same year, 26 million of Medicare's 29 million beneficiaries were age 65 and over (HCFA 1983b). Almost 10 percent of all aged enrollees

Table 6. Medicare Enrollees, Reimbursements, and Reimbursement per Enrollee, 1967–1981 *

	Enrollees (millions)	Reimbursement ($ billions)	Reimbursement per Enrolee ($)
1967	19.5	4.5	233
1968	19.8	5.7	287
1969	20.1	6.6	328
1970	20.5	7.1	346
1971	20.9	7.9	376
1972	21.3	8.6	405
1973	23.5	9.6	407
1974	24.2	12.4	513
1975	25.0	15.6	625
1976	25.7	18.4	718
1977	26.5	21.8	823
1978	27.2	24.9	918
1979	27.9	29.3	1053
1980	28.5	33.7	1184
1981	29.0	39.9	1376
	Annual Percentage Increase		
1968	1.5	25.2	23.2
1969	1.5	15.9	14.3
1970	1.8	7.5	5.5
1971	2.1	10.8	8.6
1972	2.0	9.9	7.7
1973	10.4	10.9	0.5
1974	2.8	30.2	26.0
1975	3.1	24.9	21.8
1976	2.8	30.2	26.0
1977	3.1	18.2	14.9
1978	2.7	14.5	11.5
1979	2.6	17.6	14.7
1980	2.1	15.0	12.4
1981	1.9	18.4	16.2

Sources: Calculated from HCFA 1982, p. 13, and HCFA 1983b, p.16.

*All figures include both aged and disabled enrollees.

were over age 84, up from 6 percent when the program was implemented in 1966. Sixty percent of the aged beneficiaries were women; one-third of all enrollees lived in the South, and over half lived in metropolitan areas. Medicare spending for the aged was $34.6 billion out of the total Medicare bill of $39.9 billion in 1981 (HCFA 1983b).

Growth in Medicare expenditures is caused by some of the same factors that affect the total health care system: inflation in costs, expanding technology, and increased demand for care. Medicare payments per aged enrollee have increased more markedly than health care expenditures per

Table 7. Projected Trends in Medicare Budget Outlays,* 1980–1986

	Medicare Outlays Current Law ($ billions)	Federal Health Outlays ($ billions)	Federal Budget Outlays ($ billions)	Medicare as a Percentage of	
				Federal Health Outlays	Federal Budget Outlays
FY 80 actual	35.0	58.2	576.7	60.1	6.1
FY 81 actual	42.5	66.0	657.2	64.4	6.5
FY 82 actual	46.6	74.0	728.4	63.0	6.4
FY 83 estimate	53.0	82.3	805.2	64.4	6.6
FY 84 estimate	61.5	90.6	848.5	67.9	7.2
FY 85 estimate	70.6	100.5	918.5	70.2	7.7
FY 86 estimate	79.2	109.6	989.6	72.3	8.0

Sources: OMB 1983, pp. 5–103, 6–12 and U.S. Office of Management and Budget, Executive Office of the President. 1983. *Major Themes and Additional Details Fiscal Year 1984*, p. 56.

*Outlays are for elderly and disabled and include both reimbursement for services and administrative costs.

capita, from $233 in 1967 to $1,331 in 1981, reflecting increased hospital admissions of the aged, increased services to hospitalized aged patients, and overall inflation in the cost of hospital care (HCFA 1983b).

As is shown in table 7, Medicare budget outlays are projected to increase from $35 billion in FY 1980 to close to $47 billion in FY 1982 and to nearly $80 billion in FY 1986 (OMB 1983). If the program continues unchanged, it will account for over 70 percent of projected health outlays in FY 1986, up from 60 percent in 1980; as a proportion of total budgetary outlays it will rise from 6 percent in 1980 to 8 percent in 1986.

Medicare expenditures pay primarily for hospital and physician services. As is shown in table 8, 70 percent of Medicare expenditures in 1982 paid for hospital care, nearly 22 percent for physicians' services, and less than 1 percent for nursing home care. Administrative expenses accounted for less than 3 percent of total expenditures under the program (Gibson, Waldo, and Levit 1983).

Variability among the aged in their need for and use of health care services is masked by average statistics for the program as a whole. Increased age is accompanied by increased service needs: 75 percent of those 85 or older use Medicare services compared with 70 percent of those 75–84 and 62 percent of those 65–74 (HCFA 1983b). As we have already noted, Medicare enrollees are far from homogeneous. Many are healthy and rarely use health care services. Others have multiple chronic health conditions requiring extensive care and treatment (DHEW 1978). Figure 13 shows that 7.5 percent of the aged account for over 65 percent of all Medicare

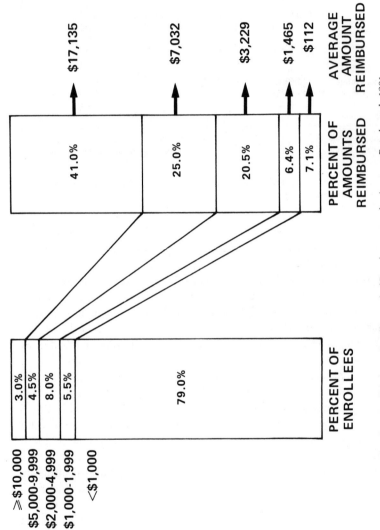

Figure 13. Percentage Distribution of Medicare Enrollees and of Reimbursements by Amounts Reimbursed, 1981
Source: HCFA 1983b, p. 45.

Table 8. Medicare Expenditures by Type of Service,* 1970, 1975, 1980, 1981, 1982
($ billions)

	1970	1975	1980	1981	1982
Total Medicare expenditures	7.5	16.2	36.7	44.8	52.2
Hospital	5.1	11.6	26.3	31.4	36.3
Physician	1.6	3.3	7.7	9.6	11.4
Nursing home	.3	.3	.4	.4	.5
Other services	.1	.3	1.2	2.1	2.7
Administrative expenses	.4	.7	1.1	1.3	1.3
	Percentage Distribution†				
Total	100.0	100.0	100.0	100.0	100.0
Hospital	68.0	71.6	71.7	70.1	69.6
Physician	21.3	20.3	21.0	21.4	21.8
Nursing home	4.0	1.9	1.1	.9	.9
Other services	1.3	1.9	3.3	4.7	5.2
Administrative expenses	5.3	4.3	3.0	2.9	2.5

Source: Gibson, Waldo, and Levit 1983.

*aged and disabled beneficiaries
†may not equal 100 because of rounding

payments for the aged. One quarter of all expenditures are incurred by the 1 percent of the beneficiaries who have average payments in excess of $15,000. At the other extreme, 38 percent of the aged receive no Medicare-reimbursed services, and another 41 percent account for only 7 percent of the payments (HCFA 1983b).

A large share of Medicare's dollars is spent for dying beneficiaries, a fact that reflects the program's coverage of the elderly. About 65 percent of those who die in a given year are Medicare enrollees. Not surprisingly, such people were more likely than others to have required health care services during the year. As a result Medicare spent $3,351 per dying person in 1976 during the last 12 months of the person's life, compared with $509 per other enrollee. Decedents represented 6.4 percent of enrollees, and Medicare expenditures in their last 12 months of life accounted for 31 percent of Medicare payments. These beneficiaries were much more likely to be hospitalized: 75 percent of decedents and 19 percent of survivors had hospital stays in a 12-month period. Average stays of decedents were slightly longer—13.8 days compared with 10.4 days. Since the cause of death of 75 percent of decedents over age 65 is heart disease, cancer, or cerebrovascular disease, a hospital episode in the last 12 months of life is probably to be expected (Lubitz, Gornick, and Prihoda 1981).

A recent study shows that Medicare enrollees who died in 1979 accounted for 5 percent of all aged Medicare beneficiaries but received close to 21 percent of all Medicare reimbursements. Approximately 28 percent of those who died received over $5,000 in services, compared with 4 percent of surviving enrollees. However, not all decedents use expensive services. One-quarter of the enrollees who died in 1979 used less than $100 in Medicare reimbursements (Helbing 1983).

It is clear that Medicare provides assistance to the elderly in the face of death and to those with serious health care problems as well as to those facing routine medical problems. Recent studies show a small proportion of the elderly are repeat and high utilizers of the program (McCall and Wai 1983; Anderson and Knickman 1984). Although Medicare is undoubtedly important for the elderly with routine medical problems, the bulk of expenditures are concentrated on a minority of the aged with life-threatening or serious chronic conditions.

Medicare's Accomplishments

Much of the impetus for the Medicare program came from the desire to lighten the burden of medical expenses for the aged. The 1963 Social Security Survey of the Aged documented that about one-half had no private health insurance (Merriam 1964). As individuals retired, they lost their employer group health insurance. Companies were reluctant to write individual comprehensive policies for the elderly for fear that they would insure an excessive number of poor risks. Available policies often limited coverage, exempted preexisting conditions, and in general offered inadequate protection. Thus remedying the failure of the private market to provide adequate health insurance was the chief goal of the Medicare program.

Medicare has clearly been highly successful in meeting this goal. It has extended health insurance coverage to virtually all elderly Americans and provided comprehensive coverage, at least for hospital services and to a lesser extent for physicians' services. Without Medicare, it is clear that medical bills for the 10–20 percent of the elderly with serious health problems would be a devastating financial burden on them and their families.

Although the primary objective of Medicare was to protect the aged against the possibility of large medical outlays, the program was also concerned with eliminating the financial barriers that discourage the elderly from seeking medical care. Since the enactment of Medicare, access to health care services for the elderly has increased substantially. In 1958, 32 percent of the elderly did not see a physician. This was reduced to 24 percent by 1970 and to 21 percent by 1976 (Aday, Anderson, and Fleming 1980).

Medicare also resulted in a major increase in utilization of hospital services by the elderly. As we noted in chapter 1, hospital admission rates climbed steeply in the first years of the program, leveled off during 1969–71, and have climbed steadily ever since. Medicare was particularly instrumental in improving access to hospital care for vulnerable elderly who were in greatest need of care—the poor, minorities, and residents of rural areas (Lowenstein 1971). Several authors have noted the impact of the program on the quality of life of the elderly, through better access to such surgical procedures as cataract operations and hip replacements (Drake 1978; Donabedian 1976).

The objectives of Medicare were concerned primarily with the financial burden of health care and assuring access to care, yet studies do confirm that the health of the elderly improved after the program's introduction. Friedman (1976), for example, found that they had fewer days of restricted activity and that this decline was inversely related to the level of personal health care expenditures. His study revealed that the mortality rates of elderly males in 1969 were lower than might have been predicted from experience prior to Medicare.

More recent data underscore the sharp decline in mortality among the aged since the introduction of Medicare. Chapter 1 noted the quite remarkable decline compared with the period before Medicare as well as with the experience of other industrialized countries during this time. A careful analysis of mortality experience of the elderly in the United States by Rosenwaike and colleagues concludes that the steep downward trend is a real phenomenon rather than a statistical artifact. The study notes the particularly marked declines for those over 84 and in deaths with an underlying cause assigned to cardiovascular condition and to cerebrovascular disease. Improved medical treatment for coronary heart disease and stroke is pointed to as an important contributor to this decline (Rosenwaike, Yaffe, and Sagi 1980).

Drake's work (1978) agrees with this analysis. He notes that one-third of the total increased longevity achieved by 65-year-olds in the first three-quarters of this century occurred between 1965 and 1975. Despite this decline in mortality rates, he points out, there has been no increase in disability among those surviving, and almost 70 percent of the elderly rate their health as good or excellent.

Although definitive conclusions are difficult to reach and multiple factors have undoubtedly contributed to this significant improvement in health of the elderly, it would appear that Medicare has had an impact on extending the lives and improving the health of this group of Americans.

Medicare's Present and Future Difficulties

Medicare is threatened by both a financing crisis and an increasing inability to protect the elderly and disabled against rising health care costs. Projections of Medicare outlays and revenues indicate very large future deficits in the Hospital Insurance Trust Fund and rapidly rising requirements for the Supplementary Medical Insurance Trust Fund. At the same time, financial protection for the elderly and disabled beneficiaries of Medicare is being eroded as out-of-pocket expenditures for cost sharing and uncovered services continue to grow.

Medicare is also coming under increased scrutiny because of its impact on federal spending and the overall federal budget deficit. In 1982 Medicare accounted for 6.4 percent of all federal outlays. Spending under Medicare increased at an annual rate of 17.7 percent from 1970 to 1982 and is projected to reach $112 billion by 1988 (CBO 1983). As was indicated earlier, the HI program is financed through the payroll tax, but the SMI program is financed by premium contributions and general revenues. The general revenue support of SMI has been increasing since the program's inception and represented 78 percent of SMI spending in 1982 (C. Davis 1983).

As cuts are made in other components of domestic spending, Medicare increasingly becomes a potential source of budget savings because of the size of both its spending and its annual increases. The projected deficit in the HI Trust Fund compounds the problem of rising expenditures and keeps Medicare at the top of the political and health policy agenda.

The HI Trust Fund Deficit

Projections for outlays and income show that the balances in the HI Trust Fund will be depleted by the late 1980s and that the fund will accumulate a deficit of $100 billion by 1995. These predictions assume that the restrictions on the rate of growth in hospital payments under Medicare enacted as part of the Tax Equity and Fiscal Responsibility Act (TEFRA) of 1982 and adopted in the Medicare Hospital Prospective Payment System (enacted in 1983) will be continued beyond their scheduled expiration in 1986, at a rate of increase equal to hospital market basket (an index of the prices of goods and services purchased by hospitals) plus one percentage point. If they are not extended, the cumulative deficit could reach $250 billion by 1995 (Ginsburg and Moon 1984).

The basic reason for the financial crisis in the Medicare HI Trust Fund clearly is rising hospital costs that drain the fund's reserves. Hospital expenditures account for nearly 90 percent of all HI spending; they have been steadily increasing at rates exceeding inflation in the general economy. Cost escalation and a growing number of elderly and disabled resulted in 18–20 percent annual increases in Medicare hospital expenditures prior to enactment of the TEFRA limits in 1982.

Projections of costs and contributions suggest that the financial problems of Medicare are chronic. The outlays of the HI Trust Fund are governed by hospital costs, but the fund's income depends on the earnings to which the HI payroll tax is applied. Hospital costs have been increasing and are expected to continue doing so at a much faster rate than the wage base for the payroll tax. The Congressional Budget Office estimates that hospital costs for Medicare beneficiaries will increase at an annual rate of 13.2 percent from 1982 to 1995, while covered earnings are projected to grow by only 6.8 percent annually (CBO 1983). The imbalances between the revenues derived from payroll tax contributions by employers and workers and Medicare hospital expenditures cause the HI Trust Fund deficit.

The aging population cannot take much of the blame for this situation. The increase in the number of elderly eligible for Medicare and the greater health care needs and utilization resulting from an older age distribution of beneficiaries will account for only 2.2 percentage points of the projected 13.2 percent annual increase through 1995. Higher hospital costs, however, will account for 10.2 percentage points (CBO 1983). Roughly half the increase in hospital costs is a result of inflation in the general economy, which requires hospitals to pay more for labor and supplies. The remainder of the escalation can be attributed to increases in hospital admissions and volume of services for Medicare beneficiaries and the increased use of expensive, high-technology procedures.

The growth in payroll tax revenues for the HI Trust Fund is dependent on the performance of the general economy. The recent recession increased the speed with which the fund was being depleted. Each 1 percent increase in unemployment reduced the fund's income by $1 billion in 1984 (CBO 1983). In addition, the Congressional Budget Office's projection of 6.8 percent annual growth in earnings assumes moderate growth for the economy in the next decade. A weak recovery or a worsening economy will exacerbate the HI financing problems by diminishing the earnings pool that is tapped to generate income for the trust fund. Even a vibrant economy, however, would not generate sufficient payroll tax income to match rising hospital expenditures over the next 50 years.

Rising Costs for the SMI Program

The SMI Trust Fund does not face the same solvency problems as the HI Trust Fund because it has a more flexible financing structure. SMI funds come from the premiums paid by beneficiaries and appropriations from federal general revenues. The law requires that general revenues be appropriated to finance all benefit and administrative costs not covered by the income from premiums. Thus the financing of the SMI program is more open ended than that of the HI fund.

Although the SMI program faces no immediate funding crisis, its increasing outlays and growing reliance on general revenue financing are of concern. SMI outlays account for one-third of total Medicare expenditures and are expected to increase by 16 percent per year through 1988 (Rivlin 1983). Since the 1972 amendments to the Social Security Act limited SMI premium increases to the percentage increase in cash social security benefits, the share of SMI costs covered by premiums has steadily declined. As has been indicated, premium payments in 1982 accounted for 22 percent of SMI expenditures, and general revenues paid 78 percent— $13.4 billion of the $17.2 billion in SMI spending (C. Davis 1983). As a result of recent legislative budget cuts, the premium will be set at a level that covers 25 percent of the incurred costs for 1983 through 1985. Unless the legislation is extended, the premium increases will again be tied to social security cost of living increases after 1985 and will renew the trend toward greater reliance on general revenues to finance SMI.

The general revenue requirements contribute to the national deficit and limit the availability of federal funds for other purposes. The Congressional Budget Office estimates that federal general revenues would have to increase by 17 percent per year to cover the projected rise in SMI outlays. This would result in an increase in SMI's share of total federal general revenues from 3.7 to 5.7 percent between 1984 and 1988. SMI outlays would have to be reduced by $27 billion from 1984 to 1988 if the goal is to hold the share of general revenue financing for the program at 3.7 percent (Rivlin 1983).

MEDICAID: LONG-TERM CARE AND ASSISTANCE FOR THE ELDERLY POOR

For the poorest of the elderly, Medicaid supplements Medicare and meets the cost-sharing requirements. Medicaid, however, is not focused specifically on the elderly. As figure 14 shows, persons 65 or older accounted for 15.9 percent of all Medicaid beneficiaries in 1981 and 36 percent of all expenditures. Medicaid spent $10 billion on behalf of the aged that year (HCFA 1983c).

Medicaid was enacted in 1965 to give federal assistance to the states in providing medical care to the poor. It was a companion piece of legislation to Medicare and served as a complement to that program.

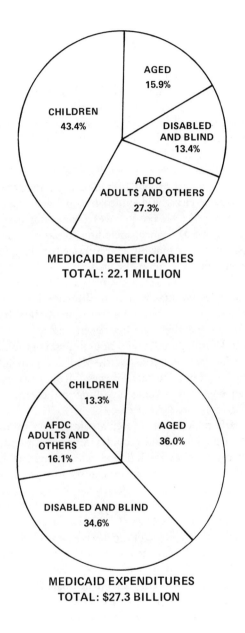

MEDICAID BENEFICIARIES
TOTAL: 22.1 MILLION

MEDICAID EXPENDITURES
TOTAL: $27.3 BILLION

Figure 14. Medicaid Beneficiaries and Expenditures by Basis of Eligibility, FY 1981
Source: HCFA 1983c, pp. 130–31.

Medicaid: The Link to Medicare

Unlike Medicare, Medicaid is a means-tested program operated jointly by the federal and state governments. Administrative responsibility and about one-half of the financial burden are borne by state and local governments. Qualifying for Medicaid is linked to eligibility for welfare and shares all the complexity and problems of that system. In the case of the elderly poor, most states cover all persons receiving federal income assistance from the Supplemental Security Income program as well as those in nursing homes.

States are required to cover several basic services under Medicaid, including inpatient and outpatient hospital care, physicians' services, laboratory and x-ray services, and skilled nursing facility and home health services. States may also choose to cover a wide array of optional services with federal matching assistance, including prescription drugs, eyeglasses, dental care, private duty nursing, and intermediate care facility services. Many, however, choose to limit the amount of a service that is covered.

Although eligibility and benefits vary widely from state to state, Medicaid remains an important source of health care financing for the poor. For the nonelderly poor it is often the only source of health care financing, and poor children and their families depend upon it to pay for primary care services and hospitalization for serious illness. For the elderly Medicaid plays a somewhat different role. With Medicare generally the primary source of financing for acute care services, Medicaid provides the elderly poor with supplementary coverage by filling in the gaps in Medicare and providing long-term care coverage.

For the elderly poor on Medicare, Medicaid pays the cost-sharing requirements and premiums and provides coverage for additional services (most notably prescription drugs, dental care, and nursing home services). For the elderly poor not entitled to social security and thus ineligible for Medicare, Medicaid provides full health care coverage.

In 1978 there were 24.7 million aged persons enrolled in Medicare SMI. Of these, 2.8 million (11.4 percent) were also covered by Medicaid under state buy-in agreements. Thus, of the 3.4 million elderly eligible for Medicaid in that year, 83.8 percent could receive Medicare through a state buy-in agreement (McMillan et al. 1983). The SMI premiums paid by the states to Medicare for these individuals totaled $282 million in 1978 and nearly $300 million in 1979 (Muse 1982).

The role of Medicaid in meeting some of the special acute care needs of low-income Medicare beneficiaries should not be underestimated, even though long-term care spending under Medicaid is much larger. Recent studies show that the dual eligibles—those entitled to both Medicare and Medicaid—are older, sicker, and more likely to be minority group members than other Medicare beneficiaries. They have higher mortality rates and higher rates of hospitalization for chronic conditions, most notably diabetes (McMillan et al. 1983). This group has 65 percent more days of hospital care and 57 percent more physician visits a year than other Medicare beneficiaries (Dobson, Scharff, and Corder 1983). For elective hospitalizations, however, such as cataract surgery, the dual eligibles and other Medicare beneficiaries have comparable rates. Their higher utilization of nonelective procedures seems attributable to greater illness rather than lack of cost sharing. Medicaid supplementary coverage for Medicare appears to provide financial access to care for the poor and frail elderly with acute as well as long-term care needs.

Trends and Variations in Expenditures

The reliance of the elderly on chronic care services, especially nursing home care, is reflected in the substantial share of Medicaid spending devoted to this group. In 1981 the average per capita expenditure per aged beneficiary was $2,921, in contrast to $930 per capita for the Medicaid population under age 65 (HCFA 1983c).

The number of aged beneficiaries has remained relatively stable over the last 10 years, but expenditures for this group have grown dramatically. In 1972, 3.3 million older Americans received nearly $2 billion in Medicaid services. Table 9 shows that by 1981, 3.5 million beneficiaries accounted for close to $10 billion (HCFA 1983c). This pattern of stable or declining numbers of beneficiaries and increasing expenditures is found for all eligibility groups under Medicaid, not just the elderly. Although the overall number of people in the program has been declining since 1977, total spending has increased from $16.3 billion in 1977 to $34 billion in 1982. It is projected that the figure will reach $48 billion by 1985 (OMB 1983).

These expenditure increases reflect Medicaid's role as a purchaser of health care services in a very inflationary market. The primary cause of Medicaid cost increases has been inflation in the health sector—not expanded eligibility or increased utilization. For example, the nearly $1 billion increase in Medicaid spending for the aged from 1980 to 1981 reflects a 3 percent increase in the number of aged beneficiaries but a 13 percent increase in expenditures (HCFA 1983c).

The Eligibility of the Elderly for Medicaid

We have noted that Medicaid eligibility for all age groups is closely linked to eligibility for cash assistance. Most Medicaid beneficiaries receive coverage automatically when they qualify for cash assistance. Aged Medicaid beneficiaries who are not on cash assistance generally qualify under op-

Table 9. Medicaid Beneficiaries 65 or Older and Total and per Beneficiary Expenditures, FY 1972–1981

Fiscal Year	Aged Beneficiaries (millions)	Expenditures on Aged Beneficiaries ($ billions)	Expenditure per Aged Beneficiary ($)
1972	3.3	1.9	580
1973	3.5	3.2	926
1974	3.7	3.7	998
1975	3.6	4.6	1291
1976	3.6	5.2	1441
1977	3.6	5.8	1619
1978	3.4	6.4	1889
1979	3.3	7.6	2283
1980	3.4	8.9	2545
1981	3.5	9.8	2786
		Percentage Change	
1973	5.4	68.1	59.6
1974	6.8	14.1	7.8
1975	−2.4	26.0	29.4
1976	0.0	11.7	11.6
1977	−0.9	12.2	12.4
1978	−6.4	10.2	16.7
1979	−2.5	19.1	20.9
1980	3.6	13.6	11.5
1981	3.0	12.9	9.5

Source: HCFA 1983c, pp. 130–31.

Table 10. Medicaid Beneficiaries and Total and per Capita Expenditures by Age and Eligibility Group, FY 1981

	Beneficiaries (millions)	Percentage Distribution	Total Expenditures ($ billions)	Percentage Distribution	Per Capita Expenditures ($)
Total, all ages	22.1		27.3		1238
Beneficiaries over 65	3.5	100.0	9.8	100.0	2786
Categorically needy	2.0	56.6	2.4	24.4	1274
Noncash categorically needy	.6	18.7	3.1	31.6	4847
Medically needy	.9	24.7	4.4	44.9	5243
Beneficiaries under 65	18.6	100.0	17.5	100.0	930
Categorically needy	15.6	83.7	12.2	69.9	816
Noncash categorically needy	1.0	5.5	1.6	9.1	1618
Medically needy	2.0	10.8	3.7	21.0	1894

Source: Calculated from unpublished statistics on Medicaid recipients and expenditures by state, FY 1981, U.S. Department of Health and Human Services, Health Care Financing Administration, Baltimore.

tional medically needy coverage offered by the state, or under special provisions allowing coverage of individuals in nursing homes. Table 10 shows the number of Medicaid beneficiaries and expenditures by age and eligibility group.

Medicaid eligibility for older Americans is predominantly shaped by federal welfare policy for the elderly. The 1972 amendments to the Social Security Act modified state discretion over Medicaid eligibility for the aged and disabled by changing the cash assistance program from a joint federal-state effort to a fully federal program called Supplemental Security Income (SSI). Almost 57 percent of the older Medicaid beneficiaries are eligible as a result of receiving cash assistance under this program. With the implementation of these amendments in 1974, the federal government assumed full administrative and fiscal responsibility for the aged, blind, and disabled welfare programs.

Under the new SSI program, a minimum income eligibility standard, applied across the country, assured comparability in welfare coverage for the poorest of the elderly. The SSI income level provides a nationwide floor for Medicaid eligibility for the aged at 74 percent of the poverty level for a single person and 88 percent of that level for a couple. In 1982 those figures were incomes of $3,408 and $5,112 per year respectively. Assets in addition to a personal dwelling could not exceed $1,500. The federal SSI income levels are indexed to the consumer price index and increase annually with inflation. Benefit levels for the elderly vary across states only to the extent that those jurisdictions wish to supplement the federal payment with more generous levels of assistance (Kutza 1981).

As was indicated earlier, some states have elected to extend Medicaid coverage to more elderly than qualify for SSI, while others are more restrictive. Table 11 shows that 32 states supplement the federal payments and provide Medicaid coverage to the elderly, who receive state cash supplements to the federal SSI payment. However, 14 states have chosen not to provide coverage to their entire SSI population (HCFA 1983a). When SSI was enacted in 1972, Congress allowed states to use their own eligibility standards that were in effect at that time instead of federal standards as a criterion for Medicaid eligibility for the aged and disabled. (Those that elected to use more restrictive standards are known as the "209 B" states.)

In addition, states may choose to cover medically needy aged. Under this option, a state can provide Medicaid coverage to persons who meet the categorical requirements for Medicaid eligibility (aged, blind, disabled, or family with dependent children), but whose incomes exceed the levels used as criteria for cash assistance and Medicaid eligibility. These people

Table 11. Medicaid Coverage for the Aged under SSI by Jurisdiction,* February 1982

Jurisdiction	All SSI Recipients	More Restricted Standard	Aged	Persons Eligible but in Institutions	Medically Needy
Total	36	14	32	42	30
Alabama	x		x	x	
Alaska	x		x	x	
Arkansas	x			x	x
California	x		x	x	x
Colorado	x		x	x	
Connecticut		x	x		x
Delaware	x			x	
District of Columbia	x			x	x
Florida	x			x	
Georgia	x			x	
Hawaii		x	x	x	x
Idaho	x		x	x	
Illinois		x	x	x	x
Indiana		x	x		
Iowa	x		x	x	
Kansas	x				x
Kentucky	x		x		x
Louisiana	x			x	x
Maine	x		x	x	x
Maryland	x		x	x	x
Massachusetts	x		x	x	x
Michigan	x		x		x
Minnesota		x	x	x	x
Mississippi	x			x	
Missouri	x		x	x	
Montana	x		x	x	x
Nebraska		x	x	x	x
Nevada	x		x	x	
New Hampshire		x	x	x	x
New Jersey	x		x	x	
New Mexico	x			x	
New York		x	x	x	x
North Carolina		x	x		x
North Dakota		x		x	x
Ohio		x		x	
Oklahoma		x	x	x	x
Oregon	x		x	x	
Pennsylvania	x		x	x	x
Rhode Island	x		x	x	x
South Carolina	x			x	
South Dakota	x			x	
Tennessee	x				x
Texas	x			x	
Utah		x		x	x
Vermont	x		x	x	x
Virginia		x	x	x	x
Washington	x		x	x	x

Table 11. Medicaid Coverage for the Aged under SSI by Jurisdiction,* February 1982 (continued)

Jurisdiction	All SSI Recipients	More Restricted Standard	Aged	Persons Eligible but in Institutions	Medically Needy
West Virginia	x				x
Wisconsin	x		x	x	x
Wyoming	x			x	

Source: HCFA 1983a, p. 84.

*Arizona does not have a Medicaid program for the elderly and disabled.

become eligible when they "spend down" by incurring enough medical expenses to reduce their available income to below the Medicaid income level. The income test for the medically needy is set by the state, but it cannot exceed 133 percent of the Aid to Families with Dependent Children cash assistance income level.

Thirty states operate medically needy programs as part of Medicaid. Nearly one million elderly Medicaid beneficiaries (one-quarter of all older persons in the program) receive their Medicaid coverage under this option (HCFA 1983a). The medically needy are the most expensive of the aged beneficiaries and accounted for 45 percent of Medicaid spending for this group. This is a product of the design of the medically needy option. First, since individuals become eligible only when their income is reduced by large medical expenses, those qualifying under this category are more likely to be sick and in need of medical services than other beneficiaries. Second, almost one-half the medically needy use nursing home services. The spend-down provision allows them to pay for part of their care with pensions and retirement funds or savings and to have Medicaid pay for the remainder.

For people who enter nursing homes with substantial resources, Medicaid coverage does not begin until all resources have been exhausted. Once that point is reached, Medicaid will cover the portion of the monthly nursing home bill that is not met by the individual's monthly social security and pension funds. This spend-down provision results in Medicaid coverage for many elderly people who were middle class until the cost of nursing home care drained their life savings and impoverished them. Thirty to 40 percent of all Medicaid nursing home residents entered as privately paying patients and later converted to Medicaid. About 60 percent of these conversions occur after the first six months of a nursing home stay (GAO 1979).

Although many of these residents qualify for Medicaid under the medically needy program, the largest group of them are eligible under special provisions for the institutionalized. States are allowed to extend Medicaid coverage to such persons with incomes below 300 percent of the maximum payment for a single person under SSI ($13,800 in 1982). This provision permits states to determine eligibility for the institutionalized aged against a higher income standard than is used for cash assistance or Medicaid coverage for the noninstitutionalized. It is an important mechanism for providing nursing home coverage in states that have not elected to cover the medically needy.

Institutional eligibility is significant because of both the growing demand for long-term care and the high cost of providing care in nursing homes. Medicaid pays for the care of over one-half of all nursing home residents. The basis for establishing someone's eligibility varies considerably nationwide, depending on whether the state covers the medically needy or uses special standards for the institutionalized.

Medicaid Benefits for the Elderly

As we explained earlier, the Medicaid program meets both acute care and long-term care needs of the elderly poor. Most states elect to provide some optional services, and virtually all offer intermediate care facility (ICF) care as an alternative to the more intensive skilled nursing facility (SNF) benefit.

Figure 15 shows that the distribution of Medicaid expenditures by type of service is significantly different for older beneficiaries. Hospital care represents over one-quarter of all spending for the general Medicaid population but less than 10 percent of that for the aged. For the latter group, the bulk of hospital expenditures is paid by Medicare, and only the deductible and coinsurance are left to be paid by Medicaid. Similarly, physician expenditures under Medicaid are small because of Medicare coverage. On the other hand, nursing home care (SNF and ICF services) is essentially uncovered by Medicare and accounts for nearly 70 percent of all spending for the aged under Medicaid (OFAA 1982).

The pattern of Medicaid spending for the elderly highlights other gaps in Medicare coverage. Prescription drugs represent a major spending item for the elderly under Medicaid. In 1981 the cost of these drugs ran to $609 million, 6.1 percent of all Medicaid spending for the elderly. Nearly 80 percent of older enrollees used the prescription drug benefit in that year (HCFA 1983a).

Utilization of various benefits under Medicaid varies by eligibility group,

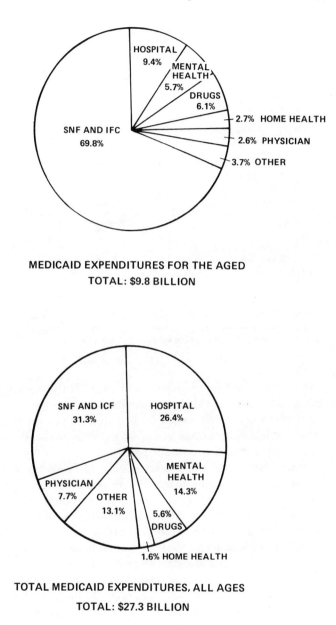

MEDICAID EXPENDITURES FOR THE AGED
TOTAL: $9.8 BILLION

TOTAL MEDICAID EXPENDITURES, ALL AGES
TOTAL: $27.3 BILLION

Figure 15. Medicaid Expenditures by Type of Service for All Beneficiaries and for the Aged, FY 1981
Source: HCFA, unpublished Medicaid statistics for FY 1981.
Note: Mental health includes care in ICF/MR.

Table 12. Use of Medicaid Services by Aged Beneficiaries by Eligibility Group, FY 1981

Type of Service	Number of Aged Using Service (thousands)	Percentage Using Services by Type Eligibility			
		All Aged	Cash Aged	Non-cash Aged	Medically Needy Aged
Acute care services					
Hospital	860	25.3	26.2	22.4	25.4
Physician	2235	65.7	68.0	63.1	62.2
Outpatient care	903	26.5	27.7	27.8	22.6
Clinic services	85	2.5	2.5	3.3	1.9
Lab and x-ray	581	17.1	14.6	18.2	21.7
Dental care	264	7.8	7.6	7.9	8.0
Prescription drugs	2663	78.3	79.6	79.4	73.9
Other	1632	47.9	44.3	41.9	60.5
Mental health					
ICF/Mentally retarded	9	0.3	0.1	0.2	0.5
Other services	53	1.6	0.7	1.7	3.5
Long-term care					
SNF	638	18.8	5.5	50.2	25.3
ICF	496	14.6	3.8	25.3	31.1
Home health	102	3.0	3.3	1.6	3.5

Source: Unpublished Medicaid statistics for FY 1981, U.S. Department of Health and Human Services, Health Care Financing Administration, Baltimore.

even among the aged. As is shown in table 12, the medically needy and non–cash assistance elderly use long-term care services far more than the aged who receive cash assistance. Less than 10 percent of the latter use a nursing home, in contrast to 75 percent of the non–cash assistance aged and 56 percent of the medically needy.

In any given year, one-quarter of older Medicaid beneficiaries have a hospital episode partially financed by the program, over 65 percent receive benefits for physician services, and nearly 80 percent receive assistance in paying for prescription drugs. The similarity in this distribution among all three categories of beneficiaries points out the use of acute care benefits financed by Medicaid for those in nursing homes.

It is estimated that Medicaid spent over $13.3 billion on nursing home services in 1982, of which $9.6 billion covered services for the aged. The money allocated to SNFs and ICFs under Medicaid understates the program's role in financing care for the nursing home population. Recent studies in New York City show that nursing home patients also consume a substantial share of Medicaid spending for acute services. During a six-month period, one-half of the nursing home residents surveyed required hospitalization and 60 percent used physician services. The average num-

Table 13. Medicaid Beneficiaries and Expenditures by Jurisdiction,* with Percentages of Expenditures for the Aged, FY 1980

Jurisdiction	Beneficiaries		Payments	
	Number (thousands)	Percentage 65 or Older	Payments ($ millions)	Percentage 65 or Older
United States, Total	21,604.4	15.8	23,301.1	37.3
Alabama	324.4	28.3	263.5	47.4
Alaska	17.2	10.7	26.7	27.5
Arkansas	222.5	28.4	234.7	42.4
California	3,417.7	16.6	2,728.2	27.4
Colorado	141.3	23.3	181.7	41.5
Connecticut	216.6	14.7	349.7	45.2
Delaware	49.2	9.5	45.3	32.2
District of Columbia	126.7	9.1	160.4	49.3
Florida	500.7	23.3	392.0	43.7
Georgia	430.3	23.6	462.4	36.7
Hawaii	106.6	10.6	96.2	35.7
Idaho	44.0	15.5	52.0	38.0
Illinois	1,048.6	7.7	1,191.9	20.2
Indiana	205.3	16.5	354.2	40.6
Iowa	178.4	18.2	230.2	41.1
Kansas	149.0	15.1		
Kentucky	410.2	18.0	295.6	32.3
Louisiana	365.2	27.3	415.2	42.2
Maine	145.6	15.4	131.3	13.3
Maryland	312.5	12.7	319.6	35.9
Massachusetts	774.9	19.9	997.9	46.3
Michigan	973.4	9.7	1,071.7	25.9
Minnesota	325.4	16.5	590.4	45.9
Mississippi	306.9	26.7	211.0	48.7
Missouri	321.5	21.4	295.1	41.6
Montana	45.8	16.2	62.3	43.3
Nebraska	71.3	21.9	108.8	44.2
Nevada	25.2	23.8	44.9	40.4
New Hampshire	44.9	21.2	71.9	61.1
New Jersey	676.3	9.2	755.9	36.7
New Mexico	87.9	13.8	70.3	26.2
New York	2,288.1	13.7	4,542.6	41.4
North Carolina	376.7	14.2	401.1	39.2
North Dakota	31.4	25.5	46.7	59.4
Ohio	808.6	15.6	809.4	33.6
Oklahoma	253.6	21.3	265.4	43.1
Oregon	277.1	11.6	178.9	30.9
Pennsylvania	1,250.6	10.2	1,058.2	34.6
Rhode Island	127.8	20.0	168.5	21.4
South Carolina	337.3	23.2	259.2	26.9
South Dakota	34.9	23.6	54.9	47.7
Tennessee	354.4	23.7	379.5	39.0
Texas	687.7	35.8	980.9	50.4
Utah	57.4	13.6	79.6	32.3
Vermont	53.8	16.4	59.3	39.1
Virginia	320.4	20.3	359.0	42.1

Table 13. Medicaid Beneficiaries and Expenditures by Jurisdiction,* with Percentages of Expenditures for the Aged, FY 1980   (continued)

	Beneficiaries		Payments	
Jurisdiction	Number (thousands)	Percentage 65 or Older	Payments ($ millions)	Percentage 65 or Older
Washington	315.2	15.4	329.0	39.8
West Virginia	129.4	15.9	103.6	29.0
Wisconsin	424.5	15.8	685.9	41.2
Wyoming	11.1	17.6	14.4	51.6

Source: Unpublished Medicaid statistics, 1981, U.S. Department of Health and Human Services, Health Care Financing Administration, Baltimore.

*Arizona does not have a Medicaid program for the elderly and disabled.

ber of physician visits per user was 8.3 during the six months. In 1980, the average cost to Medicaid per nursing home resident was $22,640, of which only three-quarters was for the nursing home per diem. The remainder was for inpatient hospital care, physician services, drugs, and related services (Storfer 1981).

The level of effort and resources devoted to the elderly under Medicaid varies among states. Table 13 shows for each state the older beneficiaries and the expenditures on their behalf as a percentage of total program beneficiaries and expenditures. The elderly constitute 15.8 percent of all Medicaid beneficiaries nationwide, with Texas having the highest proportion. Nationwide, 37.3 percent of Medicaid expenditures in 1980 were for the elderly, but the variation among states was significant—from less than 14 percent in Maine to over 50 percent in New Hampshire, North Dakota, Texas, and Wyoming (HCFA 1983a). These spending and eligibility differences reflect the different choices states have made about eligibility options, scope of benefits, and reimbursement policies.

Accomplishments of Medicaid for the Elderly

Medicaid has substantially assisted the low-income elderly covered by the program. As we have indicated, it pays for the Medicare premiums, deductibles, and coinsurance for almost three million older Americans. This reduces barriers to care and permits the use of physician and hospital services by low-income aged at a rate comparable to that of the high-income aged who have supplemental insurance coverage.

Medicaid also expands Medicare's limited benefit package to cover services that the aged poor cannot afford to purchase directly. These include prescription drugs, dental care, eyeglasses, hearing aids, and preventive services such as flu shots. Although states vary in their coverage of these services, most cover some options. Medicaid also covers some of the elderly poor people who are not covered by Medicare, such as some domestic workers and immigrants who do not receive social security.

Most importantly, Medicaid covers long-term care services excluded by Medicare and not available through private insurance. Both nursing home care and home health services are substantial components of this category. Medicaid also covers many older persons who, while not poor to begin with, become impoverished either because of the costs of chronic illness or the expenses of nursing home care.

Gaps in Coverage

Although Medicaid has done much to remedy some of the gaps in the Medicare program, it contains several inequities and deficiencies. By law, it is a program for the poor. Its long-term care benefits are available only to those who are poor or who become poor after placement in a nursing home. Its eligibility requirements, reimbursement methods, and administrative procedures frequently treat beneficiaries as second-class citizens who receive second-class care.

Furthermore, eligibility and benefit policies vary among states and result in unequal treatment of the aged. Personal care services are a relatively underused Medicaid benefit largely because of state concern over inability to control the costs of such coverage. Chore services, homemaker aid, and other types of social services have recently become eligible for Medicaid reimbursement, under a waiver provision if such benefits are shown by the state government not to increase total expenditures under the program. Implementation of this provision has been severely restricted by concern for cost.

The elderly near-poor not covered by Medicaid face the most severe barriers to obtaining care. For those who are frail, many of whom are homebound, the financial burden is especially heavy and the long-term care delivery system is often overly complex and unmanageable. Community-based long-term services are limited and poorly funded for those not eligible for Medicaid. Frequently, the needed array of services cannot be arranged and financed, and some older Americans are forced to move to a nursing home with its inclusive service package. Ironically, once in a nursing home and impoverished, the frail elderly qualify for Medicaid coverage.

LONG-TERM CARE PROGRAMS

In 1982 over $30 billion were spent in the United States on long-term care services for the elderly and disabled. Almost $1 out of every $10 spent on health care went to nursing home and other long-term care services. Nursing homes accounted for the bulk of this, with expenditures of $20.6 billion in 1981 and $27.3 billion in 1982 (Gibson, Waldo, and Levit 1983).

A little more than one-half of all long-term care services for persons of all ages were financed publicly by federal or state and local dollars. The remainder were purchased directly by consumers or their families, as there is only minimal private insurance for long-term care (expenditures in 1982 totaled only $200 million). Of the $12.2 billion in private expenditures for long-term care in 1982, $11.2 billion (97 percent) were direct payments by nursing home patients or their families (Gibson, Waldo, and Levit 1983).

Contrary to popular myths, there is little evidence that families abandon their elderly in nursing homes and leave Medicaid and the public purse to shoulder the bill. In 1976 spouses contributed an average of $2,025 to the cost of nursing home care even though their average income was only $7,890. Fewer than 10 percent of nursing home residents have a child whose income is above $20,000 (Callahan et al. 1980). Thus family support is unlikely to replace public expenditures. Almost 60 percent of all nursing home residents are publicly financed (Fox and Clauser 1980).

Despite the magnitude of public and private investment, a definition of long-term care remains one of the most elusive areas of public policy. It is difficult to define both who needs such services and exactly what constitutes long-term care. The services cover a broad range of medical, social, and supportive efforts, and the amount required varies according to the functional limitations and living environment of the person being served. There is no clearly defined line to distinguish between medical and social service needs. No single program provides the services or financing to accommodate the multiple long-term care needs of the elderly, and most are left to receive services at home from family and friends with little assistance from public programs. The lack of programs to provide support in the community can unfortunately result in placement in a nursing home for someone who can no longer cope with daily needs in his or her own home.

Public Expenditures for Long-Term Care

Public spending for long-term care has reinforced rather than reversed the incentives for institutionalization. It is estimated that in 1980 at least

$11.5 billion were spent nationally by the public sector on long-term care services, excluding the cost of care for the mentally retarded in nursing homes. Although not all of this was attributable to the elderly, that group was the major user. Nursing home and other institutional services accounted for the bulk of public expenditures for long-term care. Expenditure levels for long-term care, especially community-based care, are essentially rough estimates since the data collected generally focus on institutional care. In 1980 it is estimated that $9 billion (80 percent of all public long-term care dollars) went for nursing home institutional care (Cohen 1983).

Medicare and Medicaid, the two acute health care financing programs, are also the major public programs for long-term care assistance. Together they account for 80 percent of all public long-term care spending. Approximately 72 percent of the total was financed by Medicaid ($8.3 billion) and 8 percent by Medicare ($1 billion). Medicaid spending was largely for nursing home care, whereas Medicare spending was for home health benefits and limited SNF care. Medicaid is an important source of financing for nursing home care for the aged and accounts for 92 percent of all public spending on nursing home care. As is shown in table 14, the categorical long-term care programs, which predominantly support community-based care, pale in comparison to Medicare and Medicaid in both scope and funding. Collectively, these programs accounted for $2.1 billion in spending.

The Veterans Administration (VA) spent $460 million on nursing homes, domiciliary care, and home attendant services. Under the Title XX program, states spent $700 million on social services and other community-based long-term care support services for the elderly. The SSI program accounted for $370 million in spending for institutional care in nonmedical facilities. All other programs, including home-delivered meals and home care programs under the Older Americans Act, totaled $700 million (Cohen 1983).

Public Programs for Long-Term Care Assistance

The main public programs supporting long-term care services are Medicaid, Medicare, the nutritional and social services authorized by the Older Americans Act, Title XX of the Social Security Act, and the long-term care programs supported by the VA. Each program operates under its own rules with regard to eligibility and the provision of services. Although services or users frequently overlap, there are still serious gaps that leave many of those in need of services without care or support.

Publicly financed care is dominated by the Medicaid program, as we mentioned earlier. Under it, SNF benefits and home health services are required services. Coverage for ICF services, which provide a less intensive

Table 14. Public Expenditures on Long-Term Care Services for the Elderly and Disabled by Program, FY 1980

Service Category	Total ($ millions)	Percentage Distribution by Program					
		Medicaid	Medicare	Older Americans Act	SSI	Title XX	VA
Total	11,478*	72.2	8.1	6.1	3.2	6.3	4.1
Institutional services	9,092	87.2	3.4	—	4.1	0.2	5.1
Nursing home	8,586	92.3	3.6	—	—	—	4.1
Nonmedical facility	506	—	—	—	73.1	4.0	22.9
Community care	2,386	15.1	26.2	28.9	—	29.5	0.3
Health	775	18.2	80.8	—	—	—	1.0
In home†	668	32.6	—	6.3	—	61.1	—
Community‡	462	—	—	45.2	—	54.8	—
Meals	—	—	—	98.0	—	2.0	—
Foster care	13	—	—	—	—	100.0	—
Day care	21	3.3	—	—	—	96.7	—

Source: Calculated from Cohen 1983.

*Excludes $2 billion in ICF/mentally retarded expenditures under Medicaid since these long-term care expenditures are for the mentally retarded rather than the elderly.

†In-home services include homemaker, chore, home management, and other personal services.

‡Community services include case management, counseling, transportation aid, financial assessment, and other services.

level of care and are not required to provide 24-hour nursing, is optional but is offered by every state.

The elderly are heavy users of Medicaid nursing home services, accounting for 75 percent of such patients on Medicaid. In 1980 one million elderly people—one-third of all elderly beneficiaries—relied on Medicaid to pay their nursing home bills (HCFA 1983a). Nursing home care has thus become the middle-class component of the program.

Although Medicaid acts as a true safety net for those in nursing homes, its role in providing long-term care to needy individuals in the community is far less extensive. In 1980 some 400,000 people received $350 million of home health and personal care services from Medicaid; 35 percent of the home health care users were 65 or over. Although home health care is a required service in the Medicaid benefit package, many states provide only limited coverage. As a result, these services accounted for only 1.4 percent of all Medicaid spending in 1980. New York State dominates Medicaid spending in this regard, accounting for more than 40 percent of all home health care users nationwide and almost half of all expenditures in 1980 (HCFA 1983a).

Medicaid also covers personal care in beneficiaries' homes if a state elects to offer this benefit. It includes daily health-related activities that do not require skilled health personnel, as well as homemaker and chore services. This benefit is offered in 18 states and accounted for $217 million in Medicaid spending in 1980. New York State is again the largest spender, being responsible for 90 percent of all personal care spending under Medicaid (Cohen 1983).

Recent amendments to the Medicaid statute permit states to offer a broad range of community-based in-home services as an alternative to institutionalization. These services can be offered on a trial basis in selected areas and require federal approval prior to implementation. Experience with this provision is limited to date, but it offers a promising way to expand the scope of community services under Medicaid.

Most of the home health services provided to the elderly are financed by Medicare. However, as we described in the preceding sections, Medicare focuses on acute care and provides home health care as a follow-up to an acute illness episode rather than as a chronic care benefit. The program defines home health services as part-time or intermittent nursing care under the supervision of a registered nurse; physical, occupational, or speech therapy; medical social services; or services of a home health aide. Services must be ordered by a physician and must be delivered by a certified home health agency.

Until 1 July 1981 Medicare covered 100 visits per benefit period under

Table 15. Medicare Home Health Services, 1980

		Users		Reimbursement		
	Total Enrollees	Number (thousands)	Per 1,000 Enrollees	Total Amount ($ millions)	Per User ($)	Per Enrollee ($)
Aged beneficiaries	25,515	890	34.9	609	684	23.86
65–74	15,215	323	21.3	222	686	14.57
75 or older	10,300	567	55.0	387	683	37.57

Source: HCFA 1983a, p. 60.

the HI provisions and 100 visits per calendar year under SMI. Legislative changes enacted in 1980 knocked out all limits on the number of visits covered, eliminated the prior hospitalization requirement, and removed home health visits from the SMI deductible part of Medicare. However, the program is still restricted to recovery from acute illness. Services can be furnished only to a beneficiary who is homebound and needs either skilled nursing or speech or physical therapy occasionally.

Despite these restrictions, in recent years home health service utilization and spending under Medicare have grown significantly. Medicare expenditures increased from $61 million in 1970 to $662 million in 1980, and the number of covered visits tripled during the same period. Table 15 shows that 890,000 elderly beneficiaries used Medicare home health services in 1980. Expenditures on behalf of the elderly that year reached $609 million, 92 percent of all Medicare home health spending (HCFA 1983a).

Medicare also provides very limited coverage of care in an SNF. This is available only after a hospitalization, limited to 100 days, restricted to those requiring 24-hour skilled care, and subject to substantial cost sharing. Payment for custodial care, including help in walking or getting out of bed, is prohibited. The number of days of SNF care provided to the elderly has been declining over time. In 1970, 10.7 million days were provided; by 1980 the figure had dropped to 7.9 million days (HCFA 1983a). This decline is due to increasingly tight administrative requirements on the use of the SNF benefit (Feder and Scanlon 1982).

As is shown in table 16, in 1980 248,000 elderly beneficiaries received care in an SNF that was paid for by Medicare. The use rate for SNF services increases sharply with age, 2.7 users per 1,000 enrollees aged 65–69 to 31.2 users per 1,000 enrollees 85 or older. Because of the acute care focus of Medicare, the average Medicare-covered SNF stay was 28 days, compared with a national average of 277 days for all patients in SNFs (Cohen 1983).

Table 16. Medicare Skilled Nursing Facility Services for the Elderly, 1980

	Persons Served			Reimbursement		
	Total Enrollees (thousands)	Number (thousands)	Per 1,000 Enrollees	Total ($ millions)	Per Person Served ($)	Per Enrollee ($)
Age						
All over 65	25,104	248	9.9	331	1336	13.19
65–69	8,302	22	2.7	33	1494	3.99
70–74	6,592	37	5.5	51	1401	7.75
75–79	4,731	53	11.2	72	1356	15.22
80–84	3,072	61	19.9	80	1321	26.10
85 or older	2,407	75	31.2	95	1261	39.31
Sex						
Male	10,156	80	7.9	102	1267	10.02
Female	14,948	168	11.2	229	1369	15.33

Source: HCFA 1983a, p. 60.

The VA is an important source of long-term care services for aged veterans. It provides nursing home care, domiciliary care in VA facilities, personal care and supervision in residential care homes, and hospital-based home care. These services are administered through 172 VA medical centers located around the country. To receive care in this program, a veteran must be entitled to service-related benefits. The families of veterans are ineligible. The VA currently owns and operates 9,125 nursing home beds nationwide and contracts with private nursing homes for another 15,900 beds. About 60 percent of VA nursing home patients are elderly and nearly 90 percent are white males. In 1979 a total of 12,382 veterans received care in VA facilities, and another 28,369 were served in other facilities. The VA also operates 16 domiciliary facilities for low-income veterans with chronic impairments, generally psychiatric in nature. About one-third of the 16,602 veterans treated in these facilities are age 65 and over. In addition, the VA provides medical, nursing, social, dietetic, and rehabilitation services to homebound and nonambulatory patients. In 1980, it spent approximately $475 million on this range of long-term care services (Cohen 1983).

Some public assistance with nonmedical institutional care is provided through the SSI cash assistance program. In 1980, $370 million in SSI payments went to the support of individuals in residential care facilities (Cohen 1983). These institutional settings do not provide the medical and nursing services of a nursing home, but they do provide custodial care for the disabled and frail elderly. As we pointed out in the section on Medicaid eligibility, the SSI program is means-tested, and eligibility is limited to the aged, blind, and disabled whose income and assets are below a federally determined standard. Thus, like Medicaid, SSI benefits are available only to the elderly poor.

Title XX of the Social Security Act provides assistance to states in the financing of social services. States have considerable discretion in the design and delivery of services under this block grant. As a result, there are large variations in the eligibility criteria and the range of services covered. The extent to which the services offered emphasize long-term care depends on the preference of the state.

It is estimated that about $725 million were spent on long-term care services under Title XX in 1980 (Cohen 1983). Almost all the services under this program are community-based, since one of the major goals of Title XX is to assist individuals to achieve or maintain self-sufficiency. Many states provide homemaker and chore services for the frail elderly under this program.

The Older Americans Act is another source of funding for a wide range of community-based long-term care activities for the elderly. Financing is provided for a nationwide network of area agencies on aging that serve as advocates for the elderly and as coordination units for services. In 1980 these agencies spent $700 million (of which $570 million were federal funding) for the provision of social and nutritional services to the elderly (Cohen 1983). The services cover a wide spectrum, ranging from home-delivered and congregate meals to information and referral services. In some areas, multipurpose senior centers have been set up to serve as a coordinating point for the delivery of social and nutrition services and to provide a social and recreational center for senior citizens.

In addition to the programs described above, the federal government provides some support for congregate living facilities through the Department of Housing and Urban Development. This assistance takes the form of insured mortgages, a direct loan program, rent subsidies, and public housing aid. Funding for many of these programs has, however, been severely reduced since 1980.

Problems in the Existing System

The majority of the aged, especially those between 65 and 74, are in relatively good health and need few, if any, long-term care services. However, the prevalence of chronic illness and physical impairment among the aged, especially those over 74, means that a substantial portion of them requires some long-term care services. Roughly 1.4 million of these individuals will receive needed services in the institutional setting of a nursing home. Another 3–6 million live in the community and need community-based support services to prevent, delay, or substitute for institutionalization (Weissert and Scanlon 1983).

The existing system is frequently criticized for failure to provide adequately for the 4–7 million elderly Americans needing long-term care assistance. It is characterized by service and eligibility gaps in public programs, an inappropriate service mix, and fragmented and uncoordinated programs for the delivery of long-term care.

Eligibility gaps in existing programs create perverse incentives and can lead to impoverishment to obtain needed services. Many people are neither sick enough nor poor enough to qualify for assistance from public programs. Although the government, through Medicaid, is the largest financer of long-term care services, most older people become eligible for these only after entering a nursing home and exhausting their personal resources. The focus of programs such as Medicare on acute conditions results in the aged being unable to obtain needed services in the community to avoid institutional care.

Inflexible and often inappropriate services contribute to an institutional bias in the long-term care delivery system. One of the most obvious problems is the predominance of the nursing home as the most easily reimbursable Medicaid service. The lack of reimbursement for and availability of community-based care—such as home health, homemaker, nutrition, and chore services—often creates an incentive to use a nursing home, which can provide for all a person's basic needs. Most of the aged would not choose a nursing home over community-based care, but at the crisis stage of an illness it is often easier to obtain care in a nursing home than to develop alternatives in the home.

Nursing home supply is another serious problem faced by many of the elderly who need long-term care. Even when a person is eligible for Medicaid-reimbursed care, a place in a nursing home may not be available. A recent study found that in states with the highest nursing home bed to elderly ratio, more than 90 percent of those most in need of care (those who are unmarried, 75 years or older, and in need of assistance with all activities of daily living) were in nursing homes. In contrast, only one-half of this population was receiving nursing home care in the states with the lowest bed to elderly ratio (Weissert and Scanlon 1983).

Fragmentation among long-term care programs is an underlying cause of the inability to coordinate service packages and reimbursement in the community. The current system is a patchwork of separate public programs skewed toward the provision of either social services or health services. Rarely are the two types integrated, despite the fact that most people's needs incorporate both of these elements. Thus it is often impossible for a person's service needs to be met through a single provider or reimbursement source. Lack of effective entry evaluation and case management leaves many of the disabled and chronically ill aged without knowledge of available services and access to providers of care. Thus, even when someone qualifies for reimbursement, obtaining and coordinating services may be extremely difficult.

Long-Term Care Demonstrations

Although the United States has yet to formulate a national long-term care policy, numerous demonstration and research projects to test alternative approaches have been set up. These efforts have been aimed at overcoming the major problems of the present system—resource fragmentation, multiplicity of funding sources, and a dearth of community-based alternatives to institutional care.

The Medicare and Medicaid demonstration projects initiated during the 1970s sought to address these problems. The purpose was to identify the range of services necessary to support older people in the community and to assess the utilization and cost of such services (Lowy 1981). The development and use of needs assessment screening to divert at-risk people from institutionalization to community care was an integral component. Each person's service needs were evaluated, and a plan of care was tailored to individual requirements and family situation. A care coordinator implemented the plan by finding and arranging appropriate services in the community, monitoring the elderly person's health and social needs, and adapting the service package to meet changing needs. Medicaid or Medicare reimbursement and coverage requirements were waived to permit the coordinator to authorize payment for needed services that are normally excluded from coverage, such as transportation, homemaker and chore services, and home repair and maintenance.

The care coordinator in the early demonstrations did not serve as a care provider, but subsequent demonstration efforts are now testing this approach. Evaluation of the care coordinator's role has been inconclusive because none of these projects used a care coordinator independent of an expanded range of services (HCFA 1981).

Comparisons across sites in the early demonstration projects could not be made because of differences in research design and data collection. Most projects, however, reported that patients could be treated at lower cost in the community than in a nursing home. Although the per capita expenses were lower, expansion of services to provide comprehensive community-based care expands the user population. Many aged people, even if severely impaired, are unwilling to enter a nursing home but are willing to use services offered in the community.

These early demonstration projects could not answer policy makers' questions on the cost and effectiveness of various alternatives to long-term care delivery. The empirical evidence needed was not obtained. The unanswered research questions led to another long-term care demonstration effort by the federal government. Known as the National Long-Term Care Channeling Project, it was initiated in 1980 by the U.S. Department of Health and Human Services.

Employing a more rigorous quasi-experimental multisite research design, the new demonstration is intended to test the care coordination and expanded services model in ten sites. A common evaluation framework and standard data collection method are to be employed. Two approaches will be tested. Five sites employ a basic model using both care coordination and expanded services to provide families with needed comprehensive medical and social services not currently covered by Medicare. The other five sites use a care coordinator to provide assessment and services coordination but offer no services beyond those traditionally available under Medicare, Medicaid, or other social and health services programs.

The evaluation of the ten sites will assess the effectiveness of care coordination with and without expanded benefits. By distinguishing the impact of expanded benefits from that of the coordination of existing services, the new channeling projects should help answer questions raised by the earlier demonstrations. Researchers hope that the cost-effectiveness of alternate models can be assessed from the study results. However, as with many quasi-experimental research projects, the findings may have limited generalizability.

THE NEED FOR REFORM

Reform of the current system for financing health and long-term care services for the elderly is long overdue. Surprisingly, Medicare and Medicaid have changed little fundamentally since they were enacted. Changes have been incremental—such as addition of the disabled to Medicare in 1972—rather than through a complete reexamination of the rationale for and desirability of the current system.

A new look at Medicare and Medicaid as they affect the elderly is especially needed now. A major conflict looms between the escalating acute and long-term care health needs of a growing elderly population and economic and budgetary restraints. By 1990, as a result of the aging of the population, nursing home and hospital expenses alone are expected to consume 60 percent of all personal health care spending (Freeland and Schendler 1983). The collision course on which the United States appears to be headed indicates a clear need for prompt action. The projected deficits in the Medicare HI Trust Fund call for action to assure the financial solvency of the program.

Rather than patch things up with makeshift solutions, policy makers should view this crisis as an opportunity to design a new system that will assure the long-term adequacy and fiscal stability of financing care for the elderly. This reform should guarantee that many of our nation's most vulnerable citizens can live out their lives with dignity, freed from worry about the financial ruin that major illness can bring.

Major steps need to be taken to improve, rather than dismantle, programs that have brought many gains and achieved notable successes. In summary, the problems facing the current systems are gaps in coverage for acute care services; rising costs and projected deficits for Medicare; a growing elderly population that will increase service utilization and expenditures; means-tested Medicaid as the only source of long-term care assistance; and a long-term care system that suffers from overlapping and fragmented responsibility for services and that favors institutionalization over community-based care in its program design and eligibility policies.

Several broad strategies for reform could be pursued. Changes in financing acute care services could be dealt with separately, as is now the case, from reform of long-term care financing. Or an integrated approach encompassing both could be followed. Separate strategies are more incremental in nature and involve marginal disruption to current programs. However, they lead to gaps in meeting the needs of the elderly; contribute to fragmentation in care; distort decisions about the choice of services to meet a given health or long-term care problem; and impede innovative reimbursement policies that offer incentives for efficiency in the provision of quality health care across the spectrum of acute and long-term care services.

Whether separate or integrated financing strategies are pursued, several alternative directions are possible. The major common task is the establishment of a system to determine the allocation of resources between the health and the nonhealth sectors, between the public and private sectors, and between the elderly and the rest of the population. Possible directions include

○ placing primary emphasis upon increasing individual responsibility for making tough choices among alternatives within limited resources.

○ putting economic pressure on health and long-term care service providers such as hospitals, physicians, and nursing homes to make decisions about who receives what services within fixed budgetary constraints.

○ committing the resources and financial budgetary support required to provide adequate acute and long-term care services to the elderly.

○ shifting responsibility for decisions regarding resource allocation from the federal government to state governments.

Choosing one or a combination of alternatives will require resolution of numerous issues that go to the heart of public policy toward the elderly. It brings us back to the basic questions raised in the Introduction: What should be individual, family, or community responsibility versus public responsibility? How should the financial burden of illness or injury be distributed? If resources must be constrained, who should make the decisions about the allocation of those resources? These issues are not easily resolved. Public policy analysis is an attempt to weigh all the relevant economic, social, cultural, and political factors.

THREE

Proposals for Reforming Medicare: A Critical Review

Medicare has been subjected to increasing scrutiny during the early 1980s. The rapid rate of increase in expenditures, the significant fraction of the federal budget devoted to the program, and the projected deficits in the payroll tax–financed portion of Medicare have led to numerous reform proposals. These have been largely concerned with cost and financing issues, although some recognition has been given to gaps and inadequacies of coverage, especially for catastrophic expenses.

CONSUMER INCENTIVES

One major approach to reforming Medicare is to give those enrolled in the program greater responsibility in paying their own health care bills, on the grounds that the elderly ought to bear a greater share of the financial burden. Some contend that the financial position of the elderly has improved and will continue to do so, thus obviating some of the societal responsibility for financing their health care. Others point to projections of the growth in the size of the elderly population relative to that of workers and claim that this will make it extremely difficult for those working to continue to assume major responsibility for the health care of the older generation.

Another rationale is that having the elderly assume more of the financial responsibility for their health care bills will lead to a more efficient allocation of resources. If the elderly are required to pay a fraction of their own bills, it is argued, they will choose to receive only those services of utmost importance.

Two major proposals have been advanced to increase consumer incentives for controlling health care costs. One would restructure the current deductibles and coinsurance provisions within Medicare to give the elderly more financial participation in hospital services but better coverage of catastrophic expenses. The other would replace the current Medicare program with vouchers for the purchase of private health insurance. Limits on increases in the value of the vouchers over time would limit federal budgetary expenditures, it is claimed, and make the elderly more sensitive to rising private health insurance premiums.

Restructuring Cost Sharing

One strategy for reforming Medicare is to impose a coinsurance rate on shorter hospital stays but provide better coverage of longer hospitalization. As we pointed out in chapter 2, currently Medicare beneficiaries pay a first-day deductible ($356 in 1984) but no additional charges for the first 60 days of hospital care in a given episode of illness. Coinsurance charges at the rate of 25 percent of the first-day deductible are assessed for each day beyond 60, and a 50 percent coinsurance of the lifetime reserve is paid after 90 days.

The Reagan administration's FY 1984 budget called for considerable change in these provisions. This proposal, the centerpiece of the health budget for the year, called for a major increase in the average payment of hospitalized patients. In addition to the deductible for the first day of hospital care, enrollees would be required to pay 8 percent of this daily rate for days 2 through 15 and 5 percent for days 16 through 60. Current limits on covered hospital days would be removed. Although this proposal was not accepted by Congress, it is likely to come up again as a possible solution to reducing projected deficits in the Medicare program. The Congressional Budget Office has outlined a number of alternative hospital coinsurance proposals (CBO 1983).

Several questions could be raised about this approach. First, how much of an economic burden would increased cost sharing place on the elderly? It was noted in chapter 2 that the elderly spent $1,132 on health care services privately in 1981, a sum that is likely to increase substantially in future years even without further legislative changes.

Under this proposal, most elderly people would face substantially greater health care bills. Seven and one-half million sick, disabled, and elderly patients would face higher payments for hospital care. Those with 60 days of care during a year would pay $1,500 in hospital charges in addition to another $1,500 in uncovered Medicare expenditures—easily totaling over $3,000 annually in out-of-pocket costs.

The major burden would be felt by the aged without supplementary private health insurance or Medicaid coverage—predominantly the elderly near-poor. One way to reduce the burden on this group would be to vary cost-sharing amounts with the income of those enrolled, as was proposed at a conference on the Future of Medicare sponsored by the Committee on Ways and Means of the U.S. House of Representatives (Hsiao and Kelly 1984). Such an approach, however, entails a considerable administrative burden on the program, would undercut the universal entitlement aspect of Medicare that provides for broad-based support, and makes the system even more difficult for people to understand and use properly.

Removing the limits on days of hospital coverage under Medicare would provide better protection to 150,000 older Americans who currently incur major health care costs. However, they would still be vulnerable to catastrophic expenses for physician charges, nursing home care, private duty nursing, prescription drugs, long-term mental health care, and other benefits uncovered or only partially covered by Medicare.

Second, would this approach reduce unnecessary hospital utilization among the elderly? A recent report on a health insurance experiment among the nonelderly population by the Rand Corporation found that cost sharing reduced admission rates to hospitals (although no effect was found on length of hospital stay) (Newhouse et al. 1981). The Rand study, however, provides no evidence on whether the reduced utilization was for essential or marginal hospital care. Nor is it clear that the results would apply to the elderly. Another study has found that older people who do not supplement Medicare with private health insurance have lower utilization of services than those who eliminate cost sharing with supplementary policies (Link, Long, and Settle 1980). Again, this study provides no evidence on whether such a change in utilization is desirable or harmful.

Recent legislation to give hospitals a strong financial incentive to reduce unnecessarily long stays is likely to prove potent enough to eliminate any marginal days of care. Incentives for patients to push for earlier discharge may be of little importance.

It is clear that the extensive supplementary health insurance purchased by the elderly would mitigate the effects of coinsurance charged by Medicare. The 1980 National Medicare Care Utilization and Expenditure Survey found that 21 percent of the noninstitutionalized elderly have Medicare coverage only, while the rest have either Medicaid or supplementary private insurance (HCFA 1983a). Medicare coverage alone is systematically greater for low-income elderly. Over 28 percent of those with incomes below $5,000 have Medicare only. In contrast, 19 percent of those with incomes over $20,000 have Medicare only coverage. Hospital coinsurance would result, for those elderly who supplement, in higher premiums but very little change in actual use of hospital services. But for those lower-income elderly unable to purchase supplementary coverage, coinsurance would pose a serious financial burden.

Analysis of the economic burden and efficiency results of coinsurance also needs to consider the extreme variability of Medicare expenditures among the elderly. As we noted in chapter 1, just 7.5 percent of the elderly account for 65 percent of Medicare expenditures for this group, whereas 79 percent of the elderly incur charges of less than $1,000 per year. Thus higher coinsurance would primarily affect a fraction of the elderly with very large expenditures. For these people little marginal effect on hospital utilization could be expected, in large part because they are sure to exceed the ceiling established under the proposal.

In short, the opportunities for improving efficiency in the use of hospital services are limited under cost-sharing proposals, and the possible economic burden on some of the elderly is quite substantial. Such proposals would essentially represent a tax on the sickest and least affluent segments of society.

Medicare Vouchers

Another approach that emphasizes consumer incentives is a Medicare voucher plan. In lieu of Medicare benefits, the elderly would be given vouchers to purchase private health insurance or enroll in prepaid health plans.

One such legislative proposal is the Voluntary Medicare Option bill introduced by Congressmen Gradison and Gephardt in October 1981. Under this proposal, beginning in 1984 an amount based on the average per capita cost of Medicare adjusted to reflect differences in disability status, age, sex, and residence would have been calculated and increased annually by the medical care component of the consumer price index. Elderly and disabled Medicare enrollees could use this amount to purchase private health insurance or sign up with prepaid health plans. Eligible plans would be required to cover those services covered by Medicare, and enrollees would be guaranteed a "maximum permissible financial participation amount." If premiums for private plans were less than the Medicare vouchers, the plans would rebate the difference to the enrollees. At the end of a year, enrollees could return to Medicare if they wanted to.

An earlier bill (Stockman-Gephardt) had similar provisions, the major differences being that, once in a private plan, enrollees could not return to Medicare, that Medicare would be abolished once participation in private plans reached 60 percent, that plans would not be required to cover all Medicare benefits, and that maximum patient out-of-pocket expenses would initially be set at $2,900 and later indexed by the GNP price deflator.

Proponents argue that vouchers would foster health care market competition. Private health insurance could be expected to have more cost sharing than Medicare, giving the elderly an incentive to use services more efficiently. Low-cost health maintenance organizations would be more attractive. Private health insurance plans would have an incentive to reduce premiums by negotiating lower provider reimbursement rates.

Criticism of this proposal centers on three concerns. First, adverse risk selection may lead insurance plans to skim off the healthy elderly, leaving the very sick, chronically ill persons to be covered under Medicare. If Medicare is then eliminated and the elderly forced into private insurance plans, those plans receiving more healthy participants would fare well while those with poor risks would face financial difficulty. Given the extreme variability in health expenditures of the elderly, private plans might try to market to the healthier population by screening on the basis of medical history or providing poor service to any high-risk elderly who enroll. Whether by design or by random chance, private plans with good risks would fare well, while those with poor risks would quickly go out of business. If poor risks remained in Medicare, the total cost of the program could well rise.

Preventing adverse risk selection would require careful calibration of the Medicare voucher amount according to the health status of the particular enrollee, but tested actuarial methods for such a process do not exist. Strict regulation of marketing, enrollment, and disenrollment practices would also be key. Experience to date provides very little evidence that marketing abuses could be prevented. Sale of Medigap supplementary insurance plans to the elderly has been rife with abuses. Preventing similar problems under the voucher plan would require regulations regarding benefits covered, cost-sharing provisions, exclusions of certain services under certain conditions, exemptions of preexisting conditions, marketing practices, financial soundness of plans, enrollment and disenrollment procedures, truth in advertising, and so forth. It would redirect regulatory activities away from health care providers and toward health insurers, with little promise of effectiveness.

Second, private health insurance costs more than Medicare. Two factors suggest that costs would be higher under private plans for the same benefits to the same risk population. Medicare pays hospitals and physicians at rates below those paid by private insurance plans. In the case of hospital care, it is estimated that Medicare payments are 17 percent below those made by commercial insurance companies. Also, Medicare administrative expenses are quite low, averaging 3 percent of benefit payments. Individual insurance policies, on the other hand, have high administrative expenses, including sales commissions, advertising, and other marketing expenses. On average, administrative expenses in such plans run 30 to 50 percent of benefit payments. Hence private health insurance companies have estimated that their costs for the same benefit package would run 35 to 40 percent higher.

Third, vouchers would not be indexed sufficiently to cover rising health care costs for the aged and disabled over time. The specific legislative proposals that have been advanced all index benefits at a rate considerably lower than the expected rate of increase in Medicare expenditures. As a result, costs borne by enrollees would increase, and these might be most burdensome for the most chronically ill elderly and disabled.

PROVIDER INCENTIVES

Another approach to dealing with rapidly rising expenditures in the Medicare program is to alter incentives to hospitals, physicians, and other health care providers in an attempt to hold costs down. Major emphasis has been placed on this strategy in the early 1980s.

Hospital Incentives

The most significant step in this regard has been enactment of a prospective payment system for hospitals under the Medicare program in 1983. Hospitals now receive a fixed amount, based in part on diagnosis, per patient. This payment system is being phased in over time and varies allowable rates with differences in wages across geographical areas. Special allowances are provided for teaching hospitals and for the exceptional cases for which there is little experience on which to base a rate.

The principal savings in the system come from limiting increases in the average payment rate over time. The initial legislation holds rises to the rate of increase in the prices of goods and services purchased by hospitals (the hospital market basket price index) plus one percentage point. This level of stringency will be maintained until 1985, at which point the secretary of health and human services will be permitted to set the annual rate of increase. The limitation has an enormous impact on total Medicare expenditures. For example, if the rate of increase is set at hospital market basket plus 3.5 percentage points between 1985 and 1995, Medicare hospital expenditures will be about $150 billion higher than if the rate is held to hospital market basket plus 1 percent.

This new system, sometimes referred to as the diagnosis-related group (DRG) prospective payment system, should radically alter incentives for hospitals. For the first time a hospital that keeps patients for an unnecessarily long time, that orders an excessive number of tests, or that provides care less efficiently will be penalized. Under the previous cost-based reimbursement system, hospitals were paid more the more they did or the higher their costs turned out to be.

It is likely that the new system will need to be modified over time. At present it applies only to hospital services received by Medicare enrollees. In the short term, hospitals will have an incentive to avoid genuine cost restraint by charging privately insured patients higher rates. If hospitals are paid less for the care of Medicare patients than nonelderly patients, and if Medicare payment rates increase at a much slower rate than hospitals can collect from other patients, the disparity in payments between Medicare and non-Medicare patients could become quite marked after some time. As a result, hospitals would either refuse Medicare patients or provide a substandard level of care. One solution is to extend the current system of prospective payment to privately insured patients as well, a solution that would provide a greater incentive to hospitals to contain overall costs and would eliminate some of the potential for discrimination against Medicare enrollees.

Another difficulty with the new prospective payment system is that it does not eliminate—in fact, it exacerbates—the incentives for hospitals to increase the number of people hospitalized. Procedures that might formerly have been performed on an outpatient basis may now be done overnight. Patients may be discharged earlier, but readmission to the hospital for the same condition may increase. This problem is not readily solved within the DRG system. Hospitals could be paid only a fraction of the DRG rate for any increase in the number of hospital admissions over a previous period. For example, payment rates for additional admissions could be set at 40 percent of the DRG rate to reflect the marginal cost of an increased admission. However, the actual marginal cost to the hospital would be affected by trends in admissions of nonelderly patients as well. And some hospitals will admit more patients simply because they are located in an area where the elderly population is increasing in number. Admissions in a given year could reflect swings in patterns of illness, such as an influenza epidemic. Thus admissions that are a response to changed economic incentives and those reflecting other factors are difficult to distinguish. Approaches that would curb increasing admissions through either direct review or financial incentives have built-in problems.

Hospitals may attempt to shift some services to an outpatient basis. If tests are performed before a patient is admitted, for example, they can be paid for under the SMI portion of Medicare; the hospital could still receive the full DRG payment rate for the inpatient stay—yet that rate assumes that such tests would be performed while patients were in the hospital.

One long-range way to avoid some of these incentives is to develop capitation systems of payment that will reward hospitals and other providers for reducing hospitalization. However, such systems have their own limitations, the most serious being the absence of methods for adjusting the rates to take into account the actual health risk of the population covered.

Another disadvantage of the DRG system is that it does not take into account the severity of illness within a given diagnostic category. Since hospitals are paid the same rate for the relatively more difficult cases as for the easier cases within a category, they may have an incentive to refuse admission or to transfer the more complicated cases to other settings. Hospitals with a high proportion of more complicated cases will find their payment rates inadequate to cover costs, while other hospitals receive bonuses.

The new prospective payment system is to be phased in over three years. The substantial variations in hospital costs across different geographic regions, however, mean that the imposition of uniform national rates at the end of three years could create serious financial hardship for hospitals in some areas of the country. Facilities in the Northeast or North Central regions could suffer while those in the South and West could generate considerable profits (Lave 1984).

All these limitations point to the need for ongoing modification of the hospital prospective payment system. The effectiveness of the DRG system in containing overall increases in hospital costs remains to be determined. As adjustments will have to be made over time, the full fiscal impact is difficult to ascertain. Although the cost restraints imbedded in this system should solve some of the fiscal problems now projected for Medicare, future deficits nevertheless seem assured.

Physician Incentives

Few proposals have been advanced to limit increases in physician expenditures under Medicare. Yet the 16–18 percent annual increases in the SMI part of the program are becoming an increasing source of concern.

In its FY 1985 budget, the Reagan administration proposed "freezing" physician fees. This proposal, in fact, is a freeze not on physician fees but on the fees that Medicare will pay. Since physicians, unlike hospitals, are permitted to charge patients in excess of Medicare's allowable charge, elderly patients would bear the brunt of this proposal through higher out-of-pocket costs.

The Committee on Ways and Means of the U.S. House of Representatives coupled the freeze on fees with a proposal to require physicians to accept the Medicare fee for services rendered to hospital inpatients. This provision proved to be controversial and was met with entrenched opposition from the American Medical Association.

Yet it is difficult both to restrain rising expenditures and to protect the elderly from the financial burden of health care expenses without fundamental changes in Medicare physician payment and assignment policies. Currently, only slightly more than one-half of physician claims under Medicare are assigned (that is, the physician's fee is the same as the fee allowed by Medicare). On those claims for which physicians do not accept Medicare assignment, enrollees must pay the deductible under Medicare SMI, a 20 percent coinsurance, and the difference between the physician's fee and the Medicare allowable fee. For patients requiring expensive surgery or repeated care for a chronic condition, these noncovered expenses can be quite burdensome. Even for those with supplementary private coverage, the policies rarely make up the difference between the Medicare allowable charge and the physician's actual charge.

The U.S. Congress has expressed an interest in moving toward a prospective payment system, based upon diagnosis, for physicians. The legislation changing hospital payment methods included a provision calling for a study of such an approach. The Kennedy-Gephardt bill would prohibit physicians from charging more than the allowable Medicare fees. Medicare would establish a prospective payment rate for all services rendered by physicians to hospital inpatients, the fee to be paid to the hospital rather than to the physician. Hospitals would be required to make their own financial arrangements with physicians.

Etheredge (1983) has proposed converting Medicare to a preferred provider organization. This would require all physicians to decide whether or not to accept a fee schedule established by Medicare. Those willing to accept the fees would be listed as preferred providers, and Medicare enrollees would be encouraged to receive their care from such people. Physicians concerned about loss of patients and those for whom elderly patients represent a major portion of their practice load would be most amenable to such an approach.

Fox (1984) has proposed an even more stringent approach. Goals on per capita expenditures for health services, including both hospital and physician services, would be established on a geographical basis. Physicians in areas with expenditures lower than the goal would receive bonuses, whereas those with expenditures above the goal would receive reduced compensation from Medicare. This approach would give physicians an incentive to reduce unnecessary ambulatory physician services, hospitalizations, and physician services to hospital inpatients.

These proposals suggest possible ways to curb rising expenditures in the Medicare program. They promise to be a major source of debate in coming years. Clearly, any fundamental reform of Medicare must address physician cost-containment incentives as well as those for hospitals.

INCREASING REVENUES

Improvements in cost controls and incentives to health care providers to improve efficiency and eliminate unnecessary or ineffective care can greatly reduce projected deficits in Medicare's HI Trust Fund. But ensuring that Medicare can continue to provide adequate financial protection to the elderly and disabled in the face of ever-rising health care costs and a growing elderly population requires the reform of current methods of financing Medicare.

Sources of revenues that might be tapped to provide additional income to Medicare include

○ increases in the HI payroll tax on employers and employees or interfund borrowing from the Old-Age, Survivors, and Disability Insurance trust funds;

○ general tax revenues, largely from the personal income tax and the corporate income tax;

○ specific taxes, such as alcohol and cirgarette taxes or value-added taxes; and

○ premiums paid by Medicare beneficiaries.

Each of these alternatives has advantages and disadvantages and could be tapped to eliminate HI deficits or to support a combined HI-SMI trust fund.

Payroll Tax

The payroll tax is the current method of financing Medicare; past deficits have been met by raising it. It is administratively straightforward and requires no major change in the program. However, the payroll tax is regressive (that is, represents a higher fraction of total income for lower-income than for higher-income workers), both because there is a limit on taxable earnings and because interest, dividends, and rent income are not subject to the tax. The share of the federal budget financed by the payroll tax has risen markedly in recent years and is widely considered to place an excessive financial burden on workers.

Inter-fund borrowing would use payroll taxes raised to support social security pensions to relieve pressure on the Medicare HI Trust Fund. Under the 1983 social security financing plan, surpluses will be generated during the late 1980s and early 1990s. These funds could be borrowed to meet Medicare deficits. However, this is a short-term strategy. Surpluses in other trust funds will be required to meet pension payments in future years.

General Tax Revenues

The Medicare law could be modified to permit supplementation of HI payroll tax contributions with general tax revenues, or to merge HI and SMI into a single trust fund with general tax revenues meeting a greater share of combined expenditures than is now projected. Since general tax revenues come from moderately progressive personal income and corporate income taxes, this source of financing would be more equitable than increases in the payroll tax. With annual federal budget deficits of $100–$200 billion projected for the immediate future, channeling general tax revenues into Medicare would increase the pressure to reduce other government expenditures and would not contribute to lessening the overall budgetary deficit. However, some increase in funding from general revenues, especially in the longer term, is an option for consideration.

Cigarette and Alcohol Taxes

The alternative of generating revenues from new taxes, on such items as alcohol and cigarettes, has also been proposed. Such taxes would represent a higher fraction of income for lower-income Americans than for those with higher incomes and are therefore regressive. However, to the extent that consumption of tobacco and alcohol adds to health expenditures, it may be socially desirable both to deter their use through the economic disincentives posed by higher taxes and to redistribute some of the financial burden of health expenditures to those responsible for their creation (Long and Smeeding 1984).

Medicare Premiums

One approach to guaranteeing the future solvency of Medicare is to create a new trust fund that would merge the current revenues supporting both the HI and the SMI parts of the system. Currently scheduled payroll tax contributions toward the HI Trust Fund would continue to flow to the new trust fund, and the general revenues currently projected to cover SMI expenditures would be added. The premium paid now by the elderly for the SMI program, however, would be replaced by a premium for all of Medicare.

Universal entitlement to Medicare benefits would be guaranteed for all the elderly and disabled covered under current law. SMI coverage would no longer be optional. All Medicare benefits would automatically be provided to enrollees currently covered under HI and would not depend upon the ability to pay or the income of the elderly. This plan recognizes that much of the past success of Medicare derives from its universal coverage, which fosters program excellence and social solidarity. Further, it guarantees that Medicare program administration will not be encumbered with the administrative complexity of income determination or the potential for an adversarial role toward those enrolled in the program.

The new Medicare premium, unlike the current SMI premium, would be related to the income of those in the program and would be administered through the personal income tax system. The premium would be set at a level sufficient to guarantee the financial solvency of Medicare, and other measures such as stringent provider cost controls would be included. It is assumed that every effort would be made to achieve economies in Medicare through reasonable cost controls and incentives for health care providers to improve efficiency and eliminate unnecessary and ineffective care. Even with such measures, however, it seems likely that the overall premium for the program would need to increase beyond that of the current SMI premium. Yet the income-related feature of the premium would avoid undue financial hardship on the most vulnerable of the elderly and disabled. This system would provide much-needed financial relief to those elderly with incomes just above the Medicaid eligibility level who find the current SMI premium burdensome.

Each of these approaches deals with only one portion of the problems facing Medicare. None of them addresses gaps in long-term care coverage for the elderly or assures adequate benefits and fiscal stability for the elderly under Medicare. Nevertheless, many of the proposals contain possible components of a comprehensive reform.

FOUR

Strategies for Reform of Long-Term Care

Long-term care for the elderly has emerged as one of the most important and challenging social policy issues facing the United States today. Currently more than three million older people need the help of at least one person to live independently in the community (Weissert 1982). With the aging of the population, that number is expected to top five million by the year 2000 (K. Davis 1983). Substantial modifications in existing programs, coupled with new and innovative ways to reform the long-term care system, are required to meet the demands of a rapidly aging population.

Developing and implementing reforms will not be easy. There are no simple answers or noncontroversial approaches. The price of genuine reform that eases the financial burden for the cost of long-term care on the elderly and their families will be high. In 1982 federal and state expenditures in this sector exceeded $15 billion, and private spending was estimated to be at least another $12 billion (Gibson, Waldo, and Levit 1983). Yet these outlays account for neither the informal and unpaid help provided by family and friends nor the services that are needed but not obtained. Finding funds both to fill current gaps in coverage and to meet the growth in demand in the future is the major stumbling block to reform.

The various reforms of long-term care proposed over the last decade generally agree on the array of help necessary to enable the frail elderly and disabled to function independently in the community. Services ranging from transportation and chore services to skilled nursing care would be provided under almost all plans. The discord arises as reformers try to agree on the cost and the means of financing that care. What share of the financing should be borne directly by the individual receiving services or by the family? To what extent should care be provided and financed by the public sector? Underlying these questions are issues related to whether eligibility for publicly financed care should be based on income and how to avoid buying much of the care that is now provided free.

A variety of strategies for reform have been formulated and discussed over the last decade: developing private initiatives to increase savings or purchase insurance to protect against the risk of long-term care costs, turning services totally over to the state, offering comprehensive federal insurance, or developing comprehensive delivery systems.

CONSUMER INCENTIVES

In an era of looming federal deficits and intense pressure to reduce federal spending for social programs, many argue that it is not feasible for the federal government to do more in financing long-term care. However, most proponents of this view also recognize that the aging of the population and the lack of substantial community-based care as an alternative to nursing homes are problems that must be addressed.

Consumer incentives for reform offer one possible solution to financing that could minimize federal expenditures. In this approach, the elderly are encouraged to use their own funds to purchase services directly or to buy private insurance to cover the cost of care. Home equity conversions and modifications of the tax code to stimulate both personal savings and family support of long-term care also fall into this category.

Home Equity Conversion Options

Today 75 percent of the elderly own their own homes, and 80 percent have no mortgage on their property. The net home equity of older Americans is estimated to be approximately $550 billion (Firman 1983). Although the equity in their homes is substantial, most elderly homeowners cannot obtain cash on their investment without selling. Under the home equity conversion option, these people could continue to live in their homes but could use the cash value as a source of income, which could then be used to purchase home care and other long-term care services if and when the need arises.

There are two forms of home equity conversion: reverse annuity mortgages and sale/leaseback arrangements. Under the first, the older homeowner receives an annual income or annuity based on home equity but is also guaranteed lifetime tenancy. When that person dies, the organization providing the annuity receives the property as payment for the annuities. The sale/leaseback option functions similarly, except that the title to the property is transferred immediately rather than at the time of the homeowner's death. The former homeowner then rents the house back for life.

Both these options are premised on the belief that the elderly would be willing to encumber their homes in order to purchase long-term care that they could not otherwise afford. Proponents argue that nearly one-half the elderly at risk of needing health and personal care services live in single-family dwellings and that over one-half of these would be able to finance any long-term care services they needed for the remainder of their lives with home equity conversion. Furthermore, one-third to one-half of the elderly near-poor could be guaranteed payments of over $2,000 annually, based on the equity in their homes, for the rest of their days (Jacobs and Weissert 1984).

The primary advantage of this strategy is the magnitude of the income the elderly could generate to pay for long-term care without tapping the federal treasury. Over $70 billion in net home equity can be realized by the 2.25 million noninstitutionalized elderly homeowners who need help to live independently (Firman 1983). Home equity conversion offers a way for the elderly to be self-sufficient and pay for the care they need without having to sell their home and move in order to obtain the benefits.

There are several major obstacles to implementation, however. First, many of the elderly might be reluctant to participate in these innovative financing arrangements, for they view their home as a tangible resource that they can pass on to children and grandchildren and would refuse to turn it over to a bank or financial institution. Others would be concerned that they would lose their home and life savings under the plan. Second, those who did choose to take advantage of the home conversion option might elect not to use the cash for long-term care or might have more immediate needs for it. The potential gains for long-term care financing from conversions might never be realized. Third, there are regulatory and legal problems with home equity conversion. Changes in the tax code are required to implement the sale/leaseback option with favorable tax treatment.

Fourth, financial institutions must be willing to offer these conversion arrangements. To date, they have resisted. If someone outlives his or her home equity, the bank or loan company would not want to have to evict the elderly person. Financial institutions prefer that the mortgages be federally guaranteed to protect both the homeowner and the institution. In addition, the risk would need to be spread over a wide pool of elderly to assure that the plan would be actuarially sound. This would require the investment of large amounts of front-end capital that would remain tied up until the borrowers died. To obtain a projected return comparable with other investment options, many financial institutions would be willing to offer only an annuity with a current value substantially below the market value of the house at the time of conversion. This would make the offer less attractive to the elderly homeowner (Firman 1983).

The actual experience with home equity conversions to date is extremely limited. Nationally there have been 100 such transactions—70 in Marin County, California, and 30 in Buffalo, New York (Weinrobe 1984). In this limited experience, it appears that single women without heirs are most likely to use the option. The funds received have been used as an income supplement or to cope with short-term medical crises. The little information available thus far does not demonstrate whether the elderly would be willing to use home equity conversions to purchase long-term maintenance care or to buy private long-term care insurance.

Private Insurance for Long-Term Care

In 1982 less than 1 percent of the $27 billion spent on nursing home care was covered by private health insurance (Gibson, Waldo, and Levit 1983). Unlike acute care, long-term care has not developed as a private insurance market. As was noted in chapter 2, about one-half of all nursing home expenditures are covered by Medicaid and other public programs, and the other half come directly from payments by residents and their families. Although private long-term care insurance is offered today on a very limited basis, expansion of such policies is seen by some analysts as a viable approach to improving protection of the elderly against financial ruin in the event of catastrophic or chronic illness (Meiners 1983b).

In the private insurance approach, policies covering community-based as well as institutional long-term care services would be marketed and sold to the elderly, who would pay an annual or monthly premium to enroll in the plan of their choice. Like Medigap policies, which supplement Medicare's acute coverage, these policies would be purchased through commercial insurance companies or Blue Cross/Blue Shield.

The policies could be marketed on an individual or group basis and as indemnity or service benefit plans. Indemnity plans pay a fixed amount per day for care covered in the plan, whereas service benefit plans cover a specified set of benefits. Insurers generally prefer the former, in which they can fix their liability, over the latter, which are more open ended. The scope of coverage and the costs of private long-term care insurance will vary with the age distribution of the covered population, the size of the insurance pool, and the scope of benefits covered.

One prototype indemnity plan that has been suggested covers a nursing home stay of up to three years after a 90-day deductible. It is estimated that such a plan would require an annual premium of about $435 for a group policy or $543 for an individual one (so monthly premiums would range from $36 to $45). It is assumed that the elderly would purchase the insurance policy at age 65 and continue to pay for it throughout life except when they are receiving benefits. This plan would cover primarily nursing home care, but a similar policy could be developed to address in-home services (Meiners 1983a).

The 90-day deductible under this plan relates to the critical distinction between the short-stay patient and the long-stay patient who needs help with catastrophic expenses. The policy thus has a deductible of almost $3,000, the average cost of three months of care. After that is met, the proposed policy would pay $35 per day, roughly equivalent to the private-pay rate for one year of nursing home care in 1977. Since nursing home care costs have been increasing rapidly, it is assumed that the daily benefit payment under the plan would be adjusted annually for inflation.

One critical element in determining the premium level for private insurance plans is the age at which people buy coverage. Annual premiums can be reduced by encouraging people to buy when they are younger and by accepting longer deductible periods. A policy offering four years of coverage at $50 per day with a 90-day deductible period would require an annual premium of $544 if sold to someone age 65. The same policy with a 30-day deductible sold to someone age 75 would have an annual premium of more than $1,000 (Meiners and Trapnell 1984). It is therefore important to encourage early enrollment in private insurance plans to keep the premiums within the reach of most elderly people.

Advocates of private insurance view this plan as an attractive alternative to publicly sponsored long-term care coverage and believe it is affordable for the middle- and upper-income elderly. They argue that the cost of long-term nursing home care can be met through the indemnity benefit and the necessity of exhausting personal assets to become eligible for Medicaid can be avoided. Individuals with long-term care insurance are protected from having to join the means-tested Medicaid program and can pass their homes and assets on to their families. It is estimated that prior to their admission to a nursing home, 18–22 percent of Medicaid-supported residents had sufficient income and assets to purchase private insurance, if such policies had been available (Meiners 1983a).

The benefits of private insurance accrue to the government and tax-payers as well as to the people who purchase insurance. Medicaid expenditures for long-term care will be reduced if people are able to pay for their own care with insurance instead of spending down to Medicaid eligibility. Even if the nursing home stay exceeds the private insurance coverage and the elderly resident ultimately becomes eligible for Medicaid, savings in the program will have occurred from the delay in eligibility while private insurance provided coverage.

However, the development of private long-term care insurance coverage for the elderly faces several significant barriers. First, a private insurance market requires that there be a substantial group of people who recognize the risk of chronic disability and who are willing to pay for insurance coverage to protect themselves against that risk. Consumers appear to underestimate their need for long-term care and may not be willing to pay $500 or more per year in premiums, and it may thus be difficult to get those in their sixties to purchase plans. They may also be hard to market to the very old, who want comprehensive protection at reasonable rates.

Second, insurers argue that the existence of Medicaid as a safety net for those who become impoverished in a nursing home undermines the private insurance role. It is argued that many people will not purchase private insurance because they feel their tax dollars have already supported Medicaid and that the program should pay for them in return when they need nursing home care. Private insurance companies argue that they cannot and will not compete with the government-financed program (Lifson 1984).

Third, premium pricing presents serious problems. The risk of institutionalization increases with age. If premiums rise with age, the cost of coverage could be prohibitive for the older age groups most in need of coverage. It would also be difficult to set premium levels at a rate that anticipates inflation and delivery system changes over time. Continual revisions in premium levels would make the cost of coverage uncertain and could reduce consumer willingness to purchase coverage (HCFA 1981).

Fourth, the potential for adverse selection in the purchase of private coverage is another major obstacle. People most at risk would be most likely to purchase it. And since they were most at risk, they would tend to use services once insured. It would be difficult to develop actuarially sound premiums related to risk; if the premiums did in fact relate to risk, the cost might be prohibitive for most high-risk consumers. Low-risk consumers might not consider long-term care coverage worth the price and leave insurance coverage to the high-risk and costly consumers (HCFA 1981).

Lastly, most of the private plans currently available, as well as the prototype plan described above, focus on nursing home benefits (Meiners 1983b). Most elderly would prefer to remain in their own homes rather than enter a nursing home. Although the purchase of private insurance to protect against impoverishment in a nursing home would appeal to some people, most of the elderly would prefer coverage that provided assistance to enable them to remain in their own homes. Successful marketing of private long-term care insurance is likely to require inclusion of a home care component. However, the potential for increased demand induced by this coverage raises additional concern about premium costs. An attractive home care package used by many of the elderly could result in premiums that few could afford. Many insurers might be unwilling to market a home care package because it would be more desirable and therefore more heavily utilized by consumers than a nursing home care benefit (Meiners 1983a).

Although a few long-term care insurance plans are now offered in several areas of the country, it seems unlikely that the private insurance industry will become a dominant force in this field in the near future. Insurers want profits from the markets they enter. Most are hesitant to enter the long-term care market because of the uncertainty of its profitability. Undoubtedly, the experience of 10 plans that now offer such coverage will be closely monitored to assess the market potential (Meiners 1983b).

Tax Incentives for Long-Term Care

Tax incentives are another vehicle that could encourage private financing of long-term care. This approach would provide favorable federal tax treatment to those who save for their future long-term care needs or to families who care for a disabled parent or relative instead of placing the person in a nursing home.

One way to stimulate this is the creation of personal savings accounts, similar to Individual Retirement Accounts (IRAs), for long-term care. These private investment accounts, which could qualify for federal tax credits or deductions, could be used to finance in-home or institutional long-term care services.

Under one such proposal, people over 40 would be permitted to put 2 percent of their income up to an annual maximum of $1,000 in a private long-term care account. The first $250 in the account would be a tax credit and the remainder a deduction. At age 65, individuals could draw against their account to purchase long-term care from a federally defined set of services or could purchase a federally certified long-term care insurance plan. At death, any funds remaining in this account could be willed to a relative's or spouse's separate long-term care account. In addition to these tax incentives, this particular proposal also suggests expanding Medicaid coverage and raising social security benefits for those over 75 to improve the income support and community-based services available to the frail elderly (Fullerton 1982).

The advantage of an approach that relies on private investment is that it can be tailored to meet individual needs. The decision to set up a long-term care account and the choice of services purchased with it would be made by the purchaser and his or her family. Yet the requirement that account funds can be used to purchase only federally defined services or federally certified insurance plans seeks to assure that the funds subject to the tax break are actually used to provide long-term care. However, monitoring the expenditure of account funds would be extremely difficult. Selective audits could pick up some discrepancies in actual use of funds, but most spending would be beyond federal control.

Another concern with these accounts is that the tax breaks to encourage the investments would reduce the revenues to the federal government and thus be a drain on the treasury. And even with tax incentives, many of the elderly might be uninterested in this savings approach or might not have the financial resources to participate. The incentives on which the original proposal were based have also been weakened by recent tax code changes that liberalized the IRA provision. It would be difficult for an account earmarked for long-term care to compete with the new, unrestricted IRAs (Fullerton 1984).

Tax incentives have been proposed as a way not only to encourage people to save for their own long-term care needs, but also to encourage and maintain family assistance and support for the frail elderly. Tax deductions could be offered for the cost of in-home services or respite care or as additional personal exemptions for nonelderly taxpayers with older parents or relatives living in their home.

At the federal level, there is currently a tax credit of up to $2,400 for expenses related to the care of a dependent child or parent if the care was required to enable the taxpayer to work (Fullerton 1984). This credit primarily covers care of children who live in their parents' home and are easily established as dependent. Elderly parents often live apart from their adult children and therefore do not qualify. (However, even if an older parent lives with an adult child, the receipt of social security and pensions often violates the dependency rule). To use the tax system to encourage greater family support, tax policy could recognize contributions from children in separate households and allow them to deduct the contribution from their taxable income.

Proponents of this approach argue that financial incentives in the form of tax credits or deductions would reinforce and expand private support for long-term care. Others maintain that tax incentives would not stimulate new private long-term care spending but would instead just support the informal care that is already delivered free of charge and without financial incentives. Like long-term care accounts, this approach would also reduce federal tax revenues, and a large share of the tax credits would undoubtedly go to families that would have provided the care without new incentives (HCFA 1981).

Idaho has tried using tax incentives to expand family resources for long-term care of disabled children and adults. A state program enacted in 1980 provides a $1,000 deduction for the support in a taxpayer's home of each person age 65 and over. People with no tax liability receive a $100 tax credit for each elderly person supported. Unfortunately, preliminary results from Idaho appear to show taxpayers taking credit for support and care that may not be occurring (Bjornstad 1984). This experience suggests that tax incentives might be difficult to monitor and would at a minimum require extensive auditing.

Reforming the Delivery System

Underlying the private sector initiatives for long-term care financing and other options for reform is a belief that the delivery system requires restructuring in addition to improved financing. Replacing the dominant role of nursing homes with a greater emphasis on community-based care and developing a continuum of medical and social services tailored to individual needs are the primary objectives of long-term care reformers. The methods to achieve these goals do not rely on individual purchasing power in the marketplace as a way to reorient service toward fully coordinated and managed care systems.

Early attempts at reform through organizational restructuring centered on the concept of a single entry point for delivery. The Medicare and Medicaid long-term care demonstrations undertaken in the 1970s and the National Long-term Care Channeling Project demonstration started in 1980 are examples of the coordinated case management model of long-term care reform. In this approach, the case management agency provides an in-depth assessment of the long-term care services required by a person and then arranges for or provides them. The agency serves as both a facilitator in arranging services and a gatekeeper in controlling utilization.

These case management demonstrations tried to determine whether better coordination of existing benefits and targeting of services to those most in need could lessen the need for extensive new financing of long-term care services. The results do not provide clear answers. Organizational restructuring appears to be an essential component of reform, but a comprehensive continuum of care also seems to require integrated financing to fill the major gaps in existing program services.

The new generation of long-term care delivery systems builds upon the case management and channeling approach but adds integrated financing of services. Two examples of these new organizational approaches are the social/health maintenance organization and the life care or continuing care retirement community. These organizational structures can be used with any of the financing arrangements described above or could be coupled with various public financing options.

Social/Health Maintenance Organizations

The social/health maintenance organization (S/HMO) attempts to extend to long-term care the health maintenance organization (HMO) concept of prepayment for acute care. Both disabled and able-bodied adults could enroll in the S/HMO, which would provide a full range of integrated services, including both acute medical care and community-based and institutional long-term care. The services would be financed by periodic capitation payments, paid as a monthly premium by the elderly or reimbursed by Medicare or some other third-party payer. The S/HMO would be at financial risk to provide needed care and thus would have an incentive to ensure that services were delivered efficiently and in the least costly manner.

The basic premise behind the S/HMO is the voluntary enrollment of a defined elderly or disabled population and the guaranteed provision of a basic range of services on a capitation rather than fee-for-service basis. Acute medical services financed by Medicare would be coupled with long-term care services to enable one provider to meet the total needs of a frail elderly enrollee. The S/HMO would actually deliver a complete service package to its enrollees, whereas the earlier-generation case management organization only arranged for care from various providers. However, the nursing home benefit under the demonstration would be limited until experience with the need for such services could be established and incorporated into the S/HMO's rate structure (Diamond and Berman 1980).

The S/HMO concept has been developed since 1980 and is now ready to be tested. Four sites have been selected. Each site will have 4,000 enrollees, and the test is slated to run for at least three years. Enrollees will receive both acute and long-term care services from the S/HMOs; Medicare will pay the S/HMO on a fee-for-service basis for the acute medical services it covers. Savings on acute care combined with premiums and cost sharing will be used to pay for long-term care. Both Medicare and Medicaid will share the cost for people eligible for both programs. Initially, the sites plan to charge roughly $30 per month in premiums, a rate comparable to that for Medigap policies (Greenberg and Leutz 1984).

The proponents of this approach argue that the combination of prepaid capitation and centralization of responsibility for acute and long-term care will lead to a more coordinated and comprehensive services package and to the more efficient use of resources. They maintain that the integration of acute and long-term services allows the substitution of nonmedical social services for more expensive medical care. And they claim that the capitation approach will discourage use of costly institutional care and promote community-based services, resulting in overall savings to the S/HMO due to the substitution of appropriate, but less costly, care (Greenberg and Leutz 1984).

Proponents also point out that the financing and provision of long-term care today are fragmented among health, social services, and income maintenance programs. By pulling together the financing and provision of services, the S/HMO would link health care with social support needs and could offer an integrated service package with a continuum of care. As the single entry point for the full range of services a frail elderly person needs, the S/HMO could serve as both a care coordinator and a gatekeeper to control unnecessary utilization.

Another advantage of the S/HMO is that it reorganizes the delivery system for the elderly without changing their living arrangements. Elderly persons can use an S/HMO without moving into a retirement community, selling their homes, or otherwise disrupting their normal life style. Assets and homes remain untouched and can be passed on to children in accord with the older person's wishes.

The newness of this concept raises many questions. Whereas HMOs for acute care have been implemented, there is no practical experience with an S/HMO as a delivery system. The feasibility of setting prepayment rates for acute and long-term care has not been demonstrated. There are still major problems in adjusting HMO payments for acute care for the elderly to account for differences in health status. The added complexity of long-term care services would make accurate forecasting of expenditures difficult, which could translate into bankruptcy for plans at financial risk.

Another basic concern in the development of the S/HMO model is the minimum size of enrolled population needed. The target population will be small and may not produce a large enough enrollment base to ensure efficient spreading of risk and stable cash flow. Marketing to attract enrollees will be critical and especially difficult if the elderly already have established care providers whom they are unwilling to leave. The expansion of existing HMOs into S/HMOs and the conversion of current nursing homes, geriatric care centers, and hospitals into S/HMOs could help alleviate this problem (Diamond and Berman 1980).

Development of HMOs for acute care has progressed much more slowly than the supporters of the concept envisioned in 1971 when federal legislation to assist their launch was enacted. The experience of HMO expansion in acute care carries important lessons for the S/HMO initiative. Determining capitation payments for the elderly, controlling adverse selection, choosing communities for implementation of a new program, and monitoring the quality of care are all issues that have troubled the HMO industry and could impede the development of S/HMOs. To judge from the HMO experience, widespread implementation of S/HMOs should not be expected in the immediate future even if the test sites show the concept is sound and workable.

The four demonstration sites for the S/HMO experiment should help address many of the remaining questions about this approach. Valuable information will be obtained about the effectiveness of marketing techniques and the characteristics of those who elect to join. It will also provide a test for the actuarial methods required to predict capitation payments for acute and long-term care for the elderly. The full range of medical and social services required and used for a monitored population of 1,600 elderly people will be an important source of baseline data for future studies and epidemiologic investigation.

Life Care Communities

Life care communities (or continuing care retirement communities) are a relatively new concept in long-term care organization and delivery. The community is a total living environment including housing, social services, health care, and food in accord with a contract between the participant and the community. In essence, they provide social, health, and housing insurance for life for an aged person or couple in return for an entrance payment and monthly follow-up fees.

Arrangements for financing and requirements for entry vary from one community to another. The congregate living facilities provided range from independent town house or apartment units to a skilled nursing facility. Initially, the new member resides in his or her own unit. As health problems increase, the life care community provides an increased level of assistance, such as home help aides or home-delivered meals. When someone requires more skilled care, the community provides skilled nursing care in a facility within the community.

The resident pays an entrance fee as well as monthly payment in advance to cover the cost of these services. However, the fees are generally determined by the person's dwelling unit size and not by the scope of services required. Although the fees cover the cost of housing, there are no ownership rights. The funds are pooled so that individuals who require few services subsidize the care of those with expenditures exceeding their monthly fee or support those who exhaust their ability to pay each month. In principle, no one should ever be thrown out of a life care community— the assurance of guaranteed care until death is central.

In 1981 the average entrance fee to a life care community ranged from $35,000 to $65,000 (Alpha Center 1984). The average monthly fee for 1981 was $550, with most communities' fees in the $300–$900 range. Many of the first communities required the residents to turn over all assets upon entry. This practice has now largely been replaced by a sizeable entrance fee in combination with monthly premiums, which can be increased to keep pace with inflation.

Today there are about 275 life care communities serving some 90,000 elderly people (Winklevoss and Powell 1984). Many are located in California, Florida, Pennsylvania, Ohio, and Illinois. New York State law prohibits such arrangements. Currently the communities are primarily nonprofit corporations, often under church sponsorship. Only 5–10 percent are proprietary, although one-third of the nonprofit communities are in fact managed by proprietary companies (Alpha Center 1984). Indications are that this may be an area of proprietary company investment in the future.

Supporters of the life care community concept argue that this private sector approach of protecting against the unknown costs of long-term care also provides a solution to the fragmentation and institutional bias of the current system. Medicare continues to pay for acute care, and the remaining long-term care needs are covered under the life care contract. People are assured they will live independently as long as possible and will then receive support services. Acute care needs and long-term care services are integrated by the community providers despite the continued split in financing.

The continuum of care provided by the life care community is indeed one of its major selling points. In one central location, almost like a college campus, the full scope of needed services can be provided. These include nursing facility care, when needed. For someone who can no longer function at home, it is a more pleasant alternative than moving to a nursing home. In the life care community, the resident requiring skilled nursing facility care can remain in the community with spouse and friends nearby. If someone needs skilled care only temporarily, he or she can easily move back to the more independent living situation.

Yet these communities are not without problems. First, it is to the advantage of the community to market to the healthy and wealthy elderly.

They are generally very selective in admitting new residents. Restrictions are often placed on maximum age to control adverse selection by ensuring that the young, and normally healthier, elderly are admitted. Elderly residents with preexisting conditions are often ineligible for care. Thus life care is not an option for many of the elderly, especially those who are ill or poor.

In addition, many people will not want to live in a life care community since it requires physically relocating. For those who feel the need to move to a smaller place, however, a life care community may be suitable. As more communities develop, they are likely to be nearer to the current residences of the aging population and thus more attractive, since ties to the old community can be maintained.

Furthermore, many of the elderly may be reluctant to enter into an arrangement that consumes a substantial portion of their assets, leaving little to pass on to children or other relatives. Others will elect not to enter such a community on the assumption that they will live out their lives without the need for the long-term care coverage offered by the community.

The financial structure of the life care community is another major area of concern. State regulation is needed to ensure careful planning by communities in order to protect the financial security of the elderly. When a community has financial problems and cannot meet its commitments, residents can be left without food, shelter, medical care, or financial resources. For many, the entrance and maintenance fees could constitute their life savings. Residents' fees must be accurately calculated to project future costs and fund future renovations. It is estimated that 10–20 percent of the current communities will have some financial problems in the future because of inability to predict accurately future funding requirements (Alpha Center 1984).

Actuarial rates are difficult to develop because the level of residents' fees that can cover both current costs and future costs must be predicted. Estimating a future elderly population's death rates, morbidity, and care needs is far from a precise science. Turnover of residents is essential to the fiscal stability of the life care community, although longevity is one of the social goals. Financial success depends on collecting an entrance fee and then turning over the slot before the entrance fee has been drawn down by service utilization. The potential for underutilization of needed services is thus a concern with the life care community as well as the S/HMO.

The experience with life care communities is relatively new, and much is still to be learned about the feasibility and attractiveness of this approach for organizing an integrated housing, medical care, and long-term care system for elderly enrollees. Only 2 percent of the elderly are expected to reside in life care communities by 1990 (Alpha Center 1984). For people who are able to pay the participation fees and who want to live in an organized environment, this approach seems to offer reasonable security and care in the event of serious disability. More work needs to be done, however, to determine sound actuarial rates and to develop ways to extend this approach to the less affluent.

BLOCK GRANTS THROUGH THE STATES

Another broad strategy for long-term care reform is to give major responsibility for its organization and financing to the states. This approach builds upon the current state role in financing long-term care services under Medicaid. Under a block grant, each state would receive a fixed sum of money from the federal government for the provision of these services. The state would be given full responsibility for determining eligibility for the programs, the range of services to be provided, and the arrangements for delivery of care and payment for services. This approach can be implemented in combination with a private financing strategy or as an independent public sector strategy.

Comprehensive Block Grants

A comprehensive block grant strategy places the primary responsibility for the organization and provision of long-term care services on the state. In essence, each state is asked to design and implement its own system within broad federal guidelines. The federal government provides financing, but the state has to make the difficult decisions regarding institutional versus community-based benefits, program eligibility, and provider payment.

There are a number of ways the block grant approach can be carried out. The reprogramming of Medicaid long-term care dollars to the block grant is a basic feature, but federal funds from other programs, such as Title XX or the Older Americans Act, could also be consolidated with the Medicaid funding. Conditions in individual states such as the size and age distribution of the elderly population, the cost of medical or nursing home care, fiscal strength, and per capita income level could be taken into account in the block grant allocation formula. The scope of benefits to be offered could be broadly or narrowly defined at the federal level, depending on the degree of control sought over the funding. States could be required either to match the federal block grant dollars or to keep their spending for long-term care at its previous level. It is assumed that, even without a required contribution by the states, most would supplement federal funding.

The National Study Group on State Medicaid Strategies, composed of nine state Medicaid or public health directors, recently recommended this strategy (National Study Group 1984). The study group proposed that the current Medicaid program be replaced with a federally financed and administered primary care program and a state-administered continuing care program for long-term care. The state-run system would provide a full range of health and social services to functionally impaired individuals. States would receive federal financial assistance for these continuing care services through a block grant, each state's grant being based on the number of elderly, disabled, and mentally retarded at risk. The state would have full responsibility for defining eligibility for care and the range of services covered. This proposal follows the approach to Medicaid restructuring put forth by the Reagan administration in its New Federalism initiative.

From the federal perspective, the essential feature of the comprehensive block grant is that federal spending for long-term care would be capped. The open-ended funding under Medicaid would be replaced by a fixed annual appropriation for block grants to the states. Future federal spending for long-term care would be subject to direct, discretionary appropriation, and thus controllable. A critical issue in the design of a block grant proposal is obviously the level at which federal financial responsibility is capped and the provision for annual inflation adjustments in the cap level.

In return for the cap on federal long-term care expenditures, states would be allowed more flexibility than at present and could experiment with innovative approaches to the organization and delivery of services. They could adapt eligibility and services to meet local conditions and would be free to institute their own procedures for determining eligibility for institutional services or limiting access to in-home care to the very frail elderly. The experience of the various states could be instructive in defining further options for long-term care reform (HCFA 1981).

Supporters of the block grant approach maintain that states would be better than the federal government at reforming long-term care systems. Responsiveness to state and local conditions, coordination of multiple service delivery networks, and institution building within the long-term care community are more easily achieved at the state level (Hudson 1981). A block grant could improve coordination of services near the delivery point of care by fostering more citizen involvement and keeping long-term care high on the state policy agenda. It would also provide federal financial assistance to the states but allow state innovation without lengthy negotiations to obtain a federal waiver. Thus many of the excessive de-cision-making junctures between the federal and state government could be eliminated (Hudson 1980).

Finally, the block grant approach has appeal because it is midway be-tween tinkering with existing programs without major structural revisions and starting a whole new program for long-term care. Innovative state programs are possible without implementing a broad-scale national pro-gram (HCFA 1981).

There are, however, several major concerns about this strategy. Many view block grants as an abdication of the federal role in providing long-term care support to the elderly. Federal funding levels would be capped, and service design and delivery questions would be left to the states. There is no assurance that long-term care would remain a priority of the federal government. The lack of national standards for eligibility or benefits would promote variations among states and perpetuate existing inequities in the care of the elderly.

Block grants would end the entitlement to long-term care embodied in the current Medicaid program. An elderly person whose income and re-sources meet the Medicaid eligibility standards would no longer be assured coverage in a nursing home. Eligibility for care and the scope of covered benefits would be at the discretion of each state.

Another concern is that a separate block grant would further isolate long-term care from other health care services, undermining the contin-uum of care sought by long-term care reformers. Within a separate block grant, institutional providers could dominate the community-based care organizations in both dollars and political clout. As a result, home-based care could receive a smaller share of block grant funding than it now gets from Medicaid and the categorical grant programs (Hudson 1980).

A block grant would undoubtedly entail greater financial burdens and new political demands on state governments. With a fixed federal financial commitment, pressure to expand funding at the state level would be directed to state government. State leaders might be unwilling to commit additional resources to long-term care, or fiscal constraints could make service expansion illusory and leave a state government politically re-sponsible for an unpopular and unrewarding program (Hudson 1981).

On the other hand, the federal government would also be placed in a difficult position. Although federal funds would be paying for long-term care services in the states, the federal government would have no direct responsibility for the expenditure of funds. Future appropriations could be jeopardized by the lack of control over program design and accountability for program expenditures.

Block grants, then, have appeal from a federal fiscal perspective and remove the onus of responsibility for reform from the federal government. This must be balanced, however, against the problems that would arise in actual implementation. The fiscal pressures and general politics of long-term care combine to make the block grant a less than ideal alternative for addressing current problems in the long-term care system (Hudson 1981).

Community-based Service Grants

In lieu of comprehensive block grants for both institutional and noninstitutional services, limited grants for community-based services could be used to promote in-home care and the development of community-based alternatives to long-term care. In this approach, nursing home care would remain a Medicaid benefit, and Medicaid administration and financing would remain a joint federal-state responsibility. The entitlement for Medicaid would not be altered; health and social services now funded under Medicaid, Title XX, and the Older Americans Act could be consolidated in the community-based service grant (HCFA 1981).

This approach could be used to coordinate funding for existing long-term care or could be offered as a freestanding proposal to provide new funding for community-based services. A recent legislative proposal endorses the latter approach. It would establish a block grant to states to provide services for people at risk of being institutionalized unless support is available in their homes. Each state's allocation of the federal appropriation would be based on its share of the nation's elderly. States would be required to use the funds to coordinate home- and community-based services and to develop and implement procedures to identify both the elderly and disabled at risk of institutionalization and those in institutions but capable of living in the community (Senate 1983).

The advantages of the limited block grant are similar to those of the comprehensive approach. States would have the flexibility to provide the array of services deemed most appropriate and to introduce a continuum of services in the community. Such a grant would allow state-level decision making close to the delivery point of care, and states could experiment with ways to complement Medicaid long-term care services. The limited nature of the community-based service block grants would require less radical shifts in program policy and financing than the comprehensive block grant and would protect individual entitlement under Medicaid (HCFA 1981).

Limited grants raise many of the same concerns as comprehensive ones, but those concerns are minimized by the limited scope. Still, this limited scope means some of the desired benefits cannot be realized. Specifically, by failing to include nursing home care in the block grant, the limited approach cannot achieve neutrality between institutional and noninstitutional care; nursing home services would continue to be funded on a separate track (HCFA 1981). Similarly, both types of block grant fail to integrate long-term and acute care services. In addition, with the limited approach the federal government's costs for nursing home care would continue as an open-ended entitlement, substantially reducing the cost-control advantage for the federal government under a block grant. The narrowness of the limited block grant is thus both a strength and a weakness.

DISABILITY ALLOWANCES

One proposal that puts control closest to the point of delivery—with the person receiving care—is to provide the impaired elderly with a disability allowance that they can use to purchase long-term care. In essence, this is the individualized form of the block grant approach. Instead of a fixed appropriation to the state, a cash grant or voucher is given to the elderly person, who is then directly responsible for determining what services are to be purchased and for selecting and paying providers.

In this approach, eligibility would be based on a person's degree of functional impairment. The value of the disability allowance could be set at a single level for all cases or at multiple levels to provide more support to the severely impaired. The availability of informal family supports could be considered in the determination of the allowance level. An elderly person with family support could receive a lower allowance, for example, than someone living alone (Gruenberg and Pillemer 1980). Income could also be a criterion for eligibility or the allowance level.

The cash grant would be given in addition to a person's SSI cash assistance, pension, or social security income. It would be awarded to those at risk of institutionalization to facilitate the purchase of needed care in the marketplace (Farrow et al. 1982). One drawback is that there is no assurance that the person in need of long-term care will actually use the cash to purchase such services. In addition, consumers are left to fend for themselves in the marketplace with no control over quality of providers (Gruenberg and Pillemer 1980).

Under the voucher option of a disability allowance, a voucher for some dollar amount of long-term care would be given to a disabled elderly person. The amount would be set to reflect the anticipated cost of the range of services the person needed. In practice, the amount would be a capitation payment on the basis of level of impairment. The voucher would be redeemed as needed services were purchased. The consumer would have the freedom to choose care providers and arrange for services, but the voucher mechanism would assure that the disability allowance was used only for long-term care. Quality could be controlled by requiring use of qualified providers for vouchered services.

Supporters of an income or voucher approach argue that it would offer financial assistance to the impaired elderly without government interference in the selection and provision of services (Firman 1983). An additional benefit would be that costs would be determined by the level of cash support provided and therefore easier to control than payments to providers based on service utilization.

Opponents argue that the fragmentation of services in the current delivery system and the need to develop additional resources call for a more active government role. The frail and mentally impaired elderly would be particularly disadvantaged by this approach, since they would have to negotiate on their own for services. Another drawback is that the level of the disability allowance would be determined by the degree of impairment, something that is difficult to measure. Monitoring the disability allowances to assure accurate payment would be difficult (HCFA 1981). Furthermore, setting the voucher amount at a level to cover nursing home care would be too expensive. Thus this approach is suitable only for community-based care.

PUBLIC INSURANCE

Some reformers suggest that the solution to the long-term care problems faced by older Americans is to provide social insurance for such care as a universal entitlement. Just as Medicare provides insurance for acute health care, a new program could be implemented to provide long-term care coverage for the elderly. Alternatively, coverage under Medicare could be broadened to include social support and other long-term care services.

Comprehensive Long-Term Care Insurance

The comprehensive long-term care option would provide the elderly with protection against the long-term care costs not covered by Medicare, protection that the private market fails to offer. The policy would be government sponsored and financed, although the administration of benefits could be through private insurance companies. The compulsory nature means that all the elderly would be covered, which would eliminate the adverse selection problems of a private insurance strategy. The elderly could elect to purchase additional coverage privately if supplemental benefits were desired.

Under one prototype plan, an elderly person certified as disabled would be entitled to a wide array of services that could be tailored to meet his or her specific needs. A deductible of 10 percent of income and copayments on some services would be required to control utilization. Services exceeding the standard package would be available, but additional cost sharing would be required. A sliding-scale catastrophic limit on cost sharing would provide financial relief to the severely disabled. The state would cover those too poor to share costs in a manner similar to the current Medicaid buy-in for acute care under Medicare (Bishop 1980).

The cost of providing comprehensive long-term care insurance could be partially borne by the beneficiaries of services. Since the program would be separate from Medicare and since benefits would not be related to Medicare's social contract, the introduction of income-related cost sharing should not incur the political opposition that would arise if income testing were proposed for Medicare.

The advantage of a compulsory entitlement approach is that it covers all the elderly who meet the disability criterion, regardless of income, and spreads the risk across the broadest population base. Since long-term care is a principal cause of catastrophic health expenditures, universal long-term care coverage would protect the elderly against the risk of financial ruin from chronic health expenditures and nursing home care (HCFA 1981).

A public entitlement approach to long-term care would assist the frail elderly and their families, who now must bear alone the burden imposed by impairment (Pollack 1983). The program would replace the means-tested Medicaid program with an alternative available to the middle-class elderly, who would no longer have to impoverish themselves before being eligible for benefits. Avoiding the welfare stigma of Medicaid should increase the popularity of the program. It would also replace the state-determined eligibility and benefit policies under Medicaid with a national program with uniform eligibility and benefits. This would help to assure equitable treatment of all the elderly regardless of place of residence.

Expanding institutional and noninstitutional long-term care services under a financing program separate from Medicare would remove such services from the medical model and could encourage a more efficient mix of institutional and home care. A broad benefit package would at least promote the use of home-based services to avoid institutionalization.

Potential cost is the most significant drawback to this approach. Providing benefits to millions who are without coverage today would require increased federal outlays. Although management, restrictions on provider payment levels, and beneficiary cost sharing could help restrain costs, a substantial investment of new federal dollars would still be required.

A federally financed compulsory long-term care entitlement program could add $28–$50 billion in new federal outlays in 1985 alone, according to one estimate (CBO 1977). However, a large portion of the new federal expenditures would represent a shift in spending from the states to the federal government. Some of the new federal costs could be offset by requiring states to contribute an annual amount equal to what they would otherwise have spent on long-term care under Medicaid.

Since the administrative structure to manage such a program does not now exist, the administrative cost and burden would be substantial at first. Developing an effective federal system would require a long lead time for program implementation as well as a commitment for adequate staffing levels and administrative resources. This commitment could be difficult to obtain in an era of fiscal restraint and a determined executive branch policy to reduce the size of the federal bureaucracy.

Another drawback of a comprehensive entitlement program is that the real demand for services is unknown. The assistance currently provided by families cannot be accurately estimated. However, it is assumed that a significant portion of families now supporting elderly members informally would seek payment for the care they deliver or obtain formal care if it were covered by insurance. Moreover, future needs for long-term care assistance are likely to increase substantially over current levels because of the aging of the population and changes in family structure (HCFA 1981).

Finally, it is very difficult under any entitlement program to target services and limit utilization to those in need. That task would be especially difficult for long-term care because the assessment tools necessary for gatekeeping are still rudimentary (HCFA 1981). The range of services someone needs to continue living in the community is determined by physical and mental impairment as well as personal support and living environment. The degree of assistance required is often a matter of judgment.

Expansion of Medicare

An alternative to establishing a new long-term care insurance program is to broaden the scope of Medicare. Proposals for such reform generally suggest adding a Part C to the Medicare program to cover basic long-term care. Financing could be obtained from general revenues, payroll taxes, beneficiary premiums, or a combination of the three. This approach would build on the framework of the existing Medicare program, obviating the need for a new administrative structure.

One such proposal would increase publicly funded assistance to the elderly under Medicare by eliminating the current prohibition against custodial care and expanding today's benefits to improve coverage for in-home and nursing home care. A disability definition would be used to determine eligibility for the expanded benefits. The additional benefits would be financed by pooling existing long-term care expenditures under Medicaid and Title XX and by requiring cost sharing. A companion program, either as part of Medicare or on its own, would provide comprehensive assessments and coordinate placement of those needing long-term care (Somers 1982).

This approach offers the elderly a comprehensive benefit package providing a full range of health and social support services. The goal of developing a continuum of care and integrating acute and long-term care could be achieved through this model. Within a comprehensive approach, long-term care services should achieve greater stature than they would as a freestanding program. Yet combining services in this way could subject long-term care to an overly medical model (Somers 1980).

The funding to support the expanded benefits of this proposal is likely to require substantial new revenues in addition to the pooling of existing funds. Relying on cost sharing to meet the shortfall could seriously compromise the benefits of the expanded services and result in large out-of-pocket expenditures for the elderly near-poor.

An alternative approach to Medicare expansion suggested by Auerbach would create a voluntary "Medicare Plan C" for long-term care. According to this proposal, long-term health care insurance would be available in a form similar to the current SMI program under Medicare. Plan C would be financed by premiums deducted each month from social security benefits, with the premium set at the same level as the SMI premium. The premium would increase by 10 percent for each year after age 65 that the beneficiary did not join Plan C. To reduce the likelihood that someone would enroll in Plan C just before entering a nursing home, no one would be permitted to join after 70 (Auerbach 1982).

To receive benefits under Plan C, a person would have to be certified by a physician as needing long-term care. The plan would cover services not currently available under Medicare, including custodial care, and services could be provided in a nursing home, day care center, or the enrollee's home. Those delivering care would not be directly reimbursed by the plan. Instead, the enrollee would receive a monthly payment based on the age at which benefits began and on "reasonable monthly health care costs," determined by a commission. The benefit payment would begin at 20 percent of the reasonable monthly cost for those using benefits at ages 65–69 and would be phased up to 100 percent for those 85 or older.

Plan C would finance expanded long-term care benefits under Medicare and would remove for many of the elderly the fear of financial destitution resulting from chronic care. By relying on the already operating administrative framework of Medicare, this approach avoids duplication and the long start-up delays associated with a new program. It would foster self-reliance among the elderly by emphasizing personal choice of service package and providers.

On the other hand, this proposal promises much more than the financing scheme would support. The premiums would be the same as SMI premiums. However, the latter cover less than one-quarter of all SMI expenditures, and general revenues are used to cover the difference. Without such supplements, a trust fund for long-term care could become insolvent. In addition, this approach leaves the consumer of long-term care to fend alone in the marketplace without external payment or quality controls. The proposal also fails to address the problems of both the elderly who are not covered by Medicare and the low-income elderly who cannot afford to purchase the voluntary Plan C.

FIVE

An Integrated Approach to Reforming Financing of Acute and Long-Term Care for the Elderly

Reforming the financing of acute and long-term care services for the elderly should deal with several problems inherent in the current system. These include the financial burdens the elderly incur because of serious gaps in coverage and limitations on benefits, the projected deficit in the Medicare HI Trust Fund, the general problem of rapidly increasing expenditures for both hospital and physician services for the elderly, and the fragmented and inadequate coverage of long-term care today.

Each of the various proposals that have been advanced addresses some aspect of the problems in the present system. Yet they fail both to deal comprehensively with flaws in the current approach and to take advantage of trade-offs and coordination that could be achieved by a single, integrated plan. By dealing each with only one aspect of the current system, none seems likely to address the underlying problems in a satisfactory manner.

A Proposal for an Integrated Approach

A more promising approach is to reform both Medicare and Medicaid by addressing directly, in a fiscally responsible manner, their shortcomings in meeting the health and long-term care needs of the elderly. This involves rethinking the entire structure of the programs, including current eligibility provisions, benefits, financing sources, provider payment methods, administration, and the need for innovative features to reform the delivery of services.

The basic strategy endorsed here would be to merge the HI and SMI parts of Medicare into a single plan, develop a new voluntary long-term care plan as part of the program, and design a separate Medicaid program for Medicare beneficiaries that would provide wraparound protection for low-income elderly.

Coverage

The new Medicare program would cover everyone 65 or older (not just those covered by social security) and the disabled who qualify under current eligibility provisions. The new Medicaid wraparound coverage would be extended to all elderly poor, with a spend-down provision for the near-poor.

Benefits

All the current Medicare benefits would continue in the new plan, but the limits on covered hospital days would be removed. Deductible and coinsurance provisions for hospital and physician services would be continued. However, a new ceiling on out-of-pocket expenses on the part of the elderly would be incorporated, set initially at $1,500 and indexed over time with the growth in program expenditures. Expenses counting toward this maximum would include all out-of-pocket payments for hospital, physician, and other Medicare benefits, plus those for prescription drugs. Once an elderly person had paid $1,500 in a given year for these, Medicare would cover all additional expenses.

The optional long-term care plan under Medicare would cover nursing home care (in qualified SNFs and ICFs), home health services (in addition to the more limited home health benefits now available in the acute care Medicare plan), and day hospital services. These services would be subject to a 10 percent coinsurance charge and would have a ceiling on out-of-pocket costs of $3,000 annually. Elderly Americans wanting this coverage could enroll at 60, but benefits would not be initiated until the person had been enrolled in the plan at least five years. No one could enroll after age 70. The plan would be supplemented with a direct grant program to public and nonprofit community organizations to provide help at home, such as chore services and personal care services, for the functionally impaired.

The Medicaid wraparound plan would cover the cost-sharing payment required under the acute care part of Medicare for all elderly with incomes below the federal poverty level. A spend-down provision would assist those whose incomes would be reduced by out-of-pocket expenses to below the poverty level. The current Medicaid coverage of long-term care would continue as a safety net for those elderly poor unable or unwilling to obtain the voluntary long-term care coverage under Medicare.

Financing

The HI and SMI Medicare trust funds would be merged. The current HI payroll tax would be retained as a source of revenue for the new fund and

would continue at its current legislated rate. General revenues currently
projected to support SMI would be added to the fund, and the current
SMI premium would be replaced with an income-related payment. This
new Medicare premium would be set at 2.5 percent of taxable income of
the enrollees (compared with a current premium projected to be $203 in
1985, approximately 2.0 percent of income), and would be administered
through the personal income tax system. The definition of income would
be broadened, to be consistent with social security provisions for taxing
the benefits of higher-income elderly.

The new premium would be capped at $1,000 annually, so that no
elderly person would be required to pay a premium exceeding 50 percent
of the actuarial value of Medicare. A minimum annual premium of $100
would ensure that all elderly Americans made some contribution; for those
not required to pay income taxes, this minimum premium could be paid
directly to Medicare. Both the minimum and maximum premium rates
would be indexed over time with increases in program expenditures. Additional revenues for the new Medicare Trust Fund would come from
doubling the current tax on cigarettes. These funds would be earmarked
for Medicare and added to the trust fund.

Optional long-term care coverage would be available for an income-
related premium set at 4.0 percent of income for those who enroll at 60
(and increasing for those postponing enrollment), with a minimum annual
premium of $200. Federal general revenues would be used to meet any
long-term care expenditures not covered by the premium (as happens now
with the SMI section of Medicare). Categorical federal grant funds could
establish home help service programs through public or nonprofit community organizations.

The federal government would assume all the cost of Medicaid supplementation of Medicare acute care cost sharing. However, federal support
for residual Medicaid long-term care coverage for Medicare beneficiaries
would be reduced by one-half the current contribution rate. For anyone
receiving long-term care through Medicaid, rather than the voluntary
plan, Medicaid would assume the full cost—not just the coinsurance
provisions in Medicare.

Provider Payment

Improved benefits and expanded financing of acute and long-term care
would have to be coupled with stringent cost-containment measures. The
current prospective payment system for hospitals under Medicare would
be retained and strengthened. A residual all-payer hospital prospective

payment system covering privately insured patients as well as Medicare and Medicaid beneficiaries would be adopted for those states that do not voluntarily join in. A prospective payment system for physicians would be established, and physicians would be required to accept Medicare rates for services rendered to hospital patients. A prospective payment system for nursing homes would also be set up and would take into account the level of complexity involved in the care of patients with different functional impairments. Payment on a capitation basis would be encouraged for health maintenance organizations. Demonstrations covering both acute and long-term care, would be instituted to test capitation payment for nursing home patients as a basis for developing a longer-term prospective payment system.

Delivery of Services

Appropriate care would be encouraged through the assessment of patient conditions and by making long-term care benefits contingent upon necessity, as determined by qualified physicians. Profiles of practice patterns would be established for all benefits, and utilization review would be instituted for all claims falling outside accepted norms. Emphasis would be placed upon avoiding institutional care—in either hospitals or nursing homes—where possible. Preadmission assessment would be required for nursing homes. Day hospital services would be covered under the voluntary long-term care plan as an alternative to institutional care. Respite care would also be provided so that family members supporting a functionally impaired elderly person at home could have periodic breaks. Grants to public or nonprofit organizations to provide home help services would enable more of the functionally impaired elderly to remain in their homes. These services would also be based upon need and level of dependency. Volunteers in home help agencies could earn credits to be applied toward their own voluntary long-term care premiums.

Analysis of the Proposal

Several questions should be raised about any proposal to reform the Medicare program.

- o What is the likely impact of the proposal on Medicare enrollees?
- o How will the proposal be financed? What is its likely cost? And who will bear the burden of this cost?
- o How does the proposal relate to the existing system? And is it administratively feasible?

Impact on the Elderly

The proposed reform would remedy many of the most serious shortcomings in the current Medicare program. It would guarantee coverage for all the aged, regardless of income or prior work history. It provides comprehensive benefits, including care for acute and chronic health conditions and assistance in coping with functional limitations. It removes the heavy financial burden that currently falls on the elderly near-poor, those with chronic conditions requiring intermittent acute care, and those who require long-term care. The financial security and peace of mind that come from a ceiling on financial responsibilities for health care should go a long way toward meeting the elderly's most basic concern—the threat of insufficient funds to receive care throughout life.

The emphasis upon alternatives to nursing home care and on adequate financial protection should it be necessary provide important new benefits to the old. Current procedures work serious hardships on those unable to care for themselves. Financial access to long-term care services in the home or community is an important barrier at present. Only those who are impoverished can hope for some assistance from Medicaid. As a result, many middle-class elderly must enter a nursing home, exhaust their resources, and eventually qualify for Medicaid. A better alternative would be to support the person or the family to ensure that care could be provided in the home.

Financing

The proposed system of financing would guarantee simultaneously the fiscal solvency of Medicare through 1995, a more flexible approach, and improved benefits. The combination of revenues from the payroll tax, general revenues, cigarette taxes, and premiums should provide a stabler source of support than that of the current system. Furthermore, if projections prove inaccurate—for example, if provider cost controls and incentives have more or less impact on expenditures than predicted—premiums or the contribution from general revenues could be adjusted easily.

The deficit in the Medicare HI Trust Fund is projected to reach $250 billion by 1995. The proposed hospital payment limits would reduce this to $95 billion over the 1985–95 period (Ginsburg and Moon 1984). More recent estimates based on a better performance of the economy and slower inflation in health care costs lower the projected deficit further (Medicare Board of Trustees 1983). Other proposed reforms of physician payments and of incentives to promote alternatives to hospital care could be expected to reduce the deficit further. It is reasonable to expect that the cumulative deficit without expanded benefits or new sources of revenue would be about $50 billion over the 1985–95 period.

If fully implemented in 1985, the expanded acute care benefit package proposed here would add $1.5 billion to the cost of Medicare. This comes from placing a $1,500 ceiling on out-of-pocket expenditures (Gornick, Beebe, and Prihoda 1983). Over 10 years, improved benefits could add as much as $25 billion to the cost of Medicare. Thus the total new revenue required both to remove the current projected deficit and to improve financial protection for the elderly is approximately $75 billion from 1985 to 1995.

The proposed doubling and earmarking of the cigarette tax would generate $57 billion in revenue over this period (Senate 1984). The proposed Medicare premium would generate an additional $25 billion. (Each 1.0 percent of income paid in premiums generates $50 billion in revenues 1985–95; see Davis and Rowland 1984.)

The impact of an income-related premium on different groups of the elderly hinges on the specific manner in which the premium varies with income. Table 17 illustrates the distributional impact of four premiums using alternative percentages of adjusted gross income. Option 1 is a fixed premium for all Medicare beneficiaries with family incomes above $10,000. No premium would be assessed for those with incomes under $5,000. Premiums for beneficiaries with incomes between $5,000 and $10,000 would be on a sliding scale. Option 2 is a premium set at a constant percentage of adjusted gross income. The premium in Option 3 is a constant percentage of taxable income. Option 4 has a premium set at a constant percentage of tax liability—that is, a tax surcharge.

Table 17. Distributional Impact of Alternative Income-related Premiums, 1985*

| Adjusted Gross Income | Increased Revenue as a Percentage of Adjusted Gross Income | | | |
	Option 1	Option 2	Option 3	Option 4
Total	2.0	2.0	2.0	2.0
$0–4,999	0.0	2.0	0.1	0.0
$5,000–9,999	3.7	2.0	1.2	0.4
$10,000–14,999	4.6	2.0	2.0	0.9
$15,000–19,999	3.3	2.0	2.0	1.2
$20,000–24,999	2.5	2.0	2.1	1.4
$25,000 and over	1.0	2.0	2.1	2.6

Source: Calculated from the Brookings Institution's unpublished 1980 personal income tax file projected to 1985. Includes effects of the Economic Recovery Tax Act of 1981 and the Tax Equity and Fiscal Responsibility Act of 1982 but not the Social Security financing plan of 1983. Estimates for disabled are based on income of taxpaying units with members aged 65 and over.

*Each option yields $5 billion in revenues in 1985.

The fixed premium would be regressive at incomes above $10,000. In other words, it would represent a higher fraction of income for the elderly with incomes between $10,000 and $15,000 than for those with incomes over $25,000. Option 2, the premium set at a fixed percentage of adjusted gross income, is by definition a proportional tax. All older Americans would pay the same fraction of income to finance Medicare. The levy on taxable income is moderately progressive. Virtually no premium would be due from someone with an income below $5,000, but the elderly with incomes above $10,000 would all pay approximately the same proportion toward the program. Option 4, the tax surcharge, is the most progressive method of financing; those with incomes below $5,000 would pay virtually no premium; those with incomes between $5,000 and $10,000 would pay about 0.4 percent; those with incomes between $10,000 and $15,000 would pay 0.9 percent; and those with incomes over $25,000 would pay almost 2.6 percent of their income.

All the options for varying the premium with income are more equitably distributed than under a plan that would raise similar revenues from hospital coinsurance charges. With the premium approach, all elderly (except the low-income, if so specified) would share in the financial burden. According to the hospital coinsurance approach, however, only the 20 percent of the elderly who are hospitalized would contribute toward reduction of the deficit. Those chronically ill elderly could be faced with quite burdensome contributions under hospital coinsurance. Approximately one-fifth of the elderly at all income levels are hospitalized during a year; the average days of care are somewhat higher for lower-income elderly. As is shown in table 18, raising a comparable amount of revenue from hospital coinsurance would place enormous financial burdens on the low-income elderly who were hospitalized. Even if Medicaid were to assume these amounts for the 3.5 million elderly it covers, serious financial

Table 18. Distributional Impact of Hospital Coinsurance on Hospitalized Elderly, 1977 *

Income Class	Hospital Coinsurance Payments as a Percentage of Income
Total	6.4
Income below poverty level	27.1
Poverty to two times poverty level	16.2
2 to 4 times poverty level	6.2
Over 4 times poverty level	2.2

Source: Calculated from the unpublished 1977 National Survey of Medical Care Expenditures, U.S. Department of Health and Human Services, National Center for Health Services Research.

* Coinsurance set to yield $5 billion revenues.

burdens would be felt by people with incomes just above Medicaid eligibility. For example, the hospitalized elderly with incomes between the poverty level and twice the poverty level would pay 16 percent of their income. In addition, they would be likely to incur substantial nonhospital out-of-pocket expenditures. Clearly, as a tax matter coinsurance is the most inequitable form of taxation that could be assessed on Medicare beneficiaries.

Premiums, which represent a fixed contribution to Medicare, could not be expected to encourage or discourage use of health care services. Thus they would not pose a barrier to access to needed services. Hospital coinsurance, on the other hand, could reduce utilization, particularly for those elderly with modest incomes who do not purchase supplementary private insurance. Little is known about the types of hospital stay that would be eliminated. There is a very real danger that burdensome hospital coinsurance charges would deter many vulnerable elderly from seeking necessary care and quite obviously would place serious financial burdens on a chronically ill group of older Americans.

It should also be recognized that since the new premium would replace the current one (set at $203 annually in 1985), many elderly would pay less under the proposal than they do now. The elderly near-poor would pay 2.5 percent of income, with a minimum required premium of $100. Thus those with incomes below $8,000 would be paying a lower premium than at present.

Nearly all elderly would benefit financially from the requirement that physicians accept the Medicare allowable fee. Estimated savings to the elderly are $1.8 billion in 1985 from mandating assignment on physician services to hospital inpatients (HCFA 1983).

With the improved financial protection afforded by Medicare, many elderly might choose to drop quite costly Medigap supplementary private insurance coverage. An estimated $8 billion is spent for such coverage (Senate 1984).

Cost estimates of the long-term care component of this proposal are more difficult. The fiscal soundness depends upon the extent to which the coverage is obtained only by those in poor health. It seems that in fact the proposal could have appeal and that nearly all the elderly would opt for the voluntary long-term care coverage. If so, the projected premium should be roughly adequate to cover the full cost of the coverage—although the use of general revenues is proposed to pick up the balance should premium revenues fall short of outlays. Some demonstration of this proposal would provide an opportunity to estimate how elderly persons respond to the availability of such coverage.

Administrative Feasibility

Administering an income-related premium would represent a major departure from current administrative practice. Any systematic relationship of premiums to income would require administration through the personal income tax system. Even with this approach, however, certain administrative issues are raised. Low-income elderly who do not now file income tax statements would be required to do so under some variations of this proposal. Decisions would be required about the definition of income subject to tax—social security pensions, tax-exempt bond interest income, for example. The disabled receiving Medicare would need to be identified. Rules governing tax returns with both Medicare and non-Medicare family members or exemptions would need to be designed.

All these issues require resolution, but they do not represent insurmountable obstacles. Administration through the income tax system would ensure fair and effective compliance without the demeaning administrative procedures that means-tested benefits administered directly by Medicare would entail (Hsiao and Kelly 1984). Also, it would not engender the complexity and confusion that varying the benefit package with income would create.

The other provisions of the acute care proposal are relatively straightforward to implement. Current records are adequate to calculate the $1,500 ceiling on out-of-pocket expenditures, with the exception that the elderly would be required to submit verification of prescription drug outlays if total expenditures are near the $1,500 ceiling.

The long-term care administration would build on the current system. The direct grant program for home help services could use the existing network of voluntary agencies, senior citizens' groups, and community organizations to ensure the availability and delivery of needed home help services. The long-term care insurance component calls for the same administrative expertise as is required by current financing programs for the aged, and it should be possible to maintain the record of administrative efficiency demonstrated by Medicare.

SUMMARY

Medicare is extremely important in assuring many vulnerable older Americans of the necessary protection from financial hardship that major illness can bring. It is unthinkable that needed measures to ensure its financial soundness will not be taken. More effective cost controls and incentives for health care providers than those instituted to date are vital. Even with such measures, however, Medicare expenditures are likely to continue to outstrip currently expected revenues.

Relying on patient charges, such as hospital coinsurance, for health care services would concentrate payments on the chronically ill, many of whom have extremely modest incomes. Increases in payroll taxes or diversion of funds from general revenues are not promising for the next few years, given major increases in payroll taxes that have already occurred and the unprecedented deficits in the federal budget.

To ensure the financial soundness of Medicare, it seems imperative that a fundamental reform of its financing be undertaken. The proposal made here is to merge the HI and SMI portions of Medicare, with a combined Medicare Trust Fund financed by currently scheduled HI payroll taxes, general revenues currently projected to meet SMI expenditures, earmarked cigarette tax revenues, and a new Medicare premium related to the income of the enrollee. A merger of the two parts of Medicare would greatly enhance the flexibility of altering premiums or general revenue support in accordance with requirements of the program and the effectiveness of cost-containment measures, and it would simplify budgetary considerations.

Reliance upon a premium that varies with income would guarantee that any financial contribution by those receiving Medicare would be equitably borne and would not place a burden on any group or person. With an assured, stable funding base, Medicare benefits could be expanded to fill many current gaps in acute and long-term care. Coupled with provider cost controls, such as extension of current limits on hospital payments and physician fee schedules with mandatory assignment, this financing reform could restore Medicare's original promise of ensuring adequate health care for all older Americans without the threat of financial ruin.

This proposal requires careful consideration and debate. But it should not be forgotten that many of our nation's most vulnerable citizens depend upon Medicare to live their lives with dignity. These reforms would free them of the worry of financial ruin that major illness can bring while simultaneously assuring the long-term adequacy and fiscal stability of the Medicare program. In the current climate of fiscal stringency, it is important that we work to protect and improve the essential character of these programs, rather than dismantle a system that has brought much-needed protection to older Americans.

APPENDIX

The Impact of Aging on the Future Health System in the United States

The projections used in the text are taken from the Computer Assisted Planning (CAP) model developed at the Johns Hopkins University.[1] Data for it are drawn from over 200 sources, including various surveys conducted by the National Center for Health Statistics and the Health Care Financing Administration of the U.S. Department of Health and Human Services, and by the Bureau of the Census of the U.S. Department of Commerce. This data base contains current information on the demographic characteristics and socioeconomic status of Americans, the economy, labor force participation, social security, housing, social services, health services and their utilization, health status, long-term care needs and utilization, and health expenditures.

Projections for future years are based on official government estimates of the prospective population by age, sex, and race cohort. The model incorporates the Bureau of the Census's assumption of 400,000 net immigrants annually and a fertility rate of 2.1 children per woman aged 14–49. Mortality rates are based on projections by actuaries of the Social Security Administration by age, sex, race, and cause of death. These estimates predict a 36 percent decline in the age-adjusted death rate for the United States between 1978 and 2055, which is used as the official forecast by the actuaries.

Several methodologies have been used to project the impact of aging on the health care system. In areas for which extensive studies have already been done, results have been incorporated into the model. For example, projections of the physician supply are those of the Graduate Medical Education National Advisory Committee.[2]

Projections of health expenditures are based on econometric estimates by age group (65 or older, 19–64, and under 19) and by type of services (for example, hospital, physician, or nursing home) for 1965 to 1978. Log linear regression equations of per capita health expenditures yield annual growth rates in constant dollars over this historical period. The constant dollar annual growth rates are then applied to yield forecasts of per capita health expenditures by age group and type of health service.

Mortality rates by cause of death are based on estimates of actuaries of the Social Security Administration.[3] For the most part, these estimates suggest that the trends in mortality rates by age and sex of the past 15 years will continue, but at more moderate rates of increase or decline. The actuaries assume little further improvement in mortality rates from infectious diseases, continued improvement in mortality rates from degenerative diseases, and an increase in deaths from violent causes, principally among young adults.

Forecasts of morbidity levels in the U.S. population are based on the assumption that prevalence rates by age and sex cohort will stay constant over time. This is a controversial assumption. Kramer and Gruenberg, for example, argue that the seriously disabled or chronically ill are now living longer because of the success of technical innovations used in disease control. They argue, therefore, that the prevalence rate of disabling and chronic conditions will increase over time, by prolonging the average duration of such conditions.[4] Manton, on the other hand, argues that there is no evidence that the average health status of the aged has declined in recent years, despite a very dramatic decline in mortality rates of the aged.[5] In the absence of convincing evidence on this controversy, the prevalence of disability or functional limitation per person of a given age-sex cohort is assumed to be constant over time. The total level of disabling conditions in the population in the future has been determined, therefore, by the growth of population cohorts.

Given the rudimentary state of development of projection methodologies, projections—especially those far in the future—must be viewed cautiously. Technological advances could alter them considerably. Fertility rates could continue to decline markedly or could increase, greatly affecting the size of the work force supporting the aged population. Immigration from Mexico or Third World countries could take up some of the slack created by the slowing growth of the U.S. native population. Most importantly, these projections assume that current policies will continue unchanged.

The CAP model used for these projections has broader applications. One of its major purposes is to simulate the effect of alternative policies and demographic, morbidity, and mortality assumptions on the future course of the health system. The model is also in use for Canada, two Canadian provinces, and Norway. Work is currently under way to apply the model to other geographic areas in order to simulate policy alternatives being addressed by national and regional governments.

NOTES

1. CAP was developed at the Johns Hopkins University School of Hygiene and Public Health with support from the World Health Organization, European Regional Office. For further information about the projection methodologies and results, see Karen Davis, "Health Implications of Aging in America," conference on the Impact of Technology on Aging in America, sponsored by the U.S. Congress, Office of Technology Assessment, Millwood, Va., 16–18 February 1983.

2. U.S. Department of Health and Human Services, Health Resources Administration, *Summary Report of the Graduate Medical Education National Advisory Committee to the Secretary of the Department of Health and Human Services*, vol. 1, 30 September 1980.

3. U.S. Social Security Administration, Office of the Actuary, published in Dorothy P. Rice and Jacob J. Feldman, *Tables and Charts for Demographic Changes and the Health Needs of the Elderly, Perspectives in Science and Policy* (Washington, D.C.: National Academy of Science, Institute of Medicine, 20 October 1982), table 2.

4. See Ernest M. Gruenberg, "The Failure of Success," *Milbank Memorial Fund Quarterly/Health and Society*. 55 (Winter 1977): 3–24; and Morton Kramer, "The Rising Pandemic of Mental Disorders and Associated Chronic Diseases and Disabilities," in "Epidemiologic Research and a Basis for the Organization of Extramural Psychiatry," *Acta Psychiatrica Scandinavia*, Supplement 285, 62 (1980): 382–96; see also J. F. Fries, "Aging, Natural Death and the Compression of Morbidity," *New England Journal of Medicine* 303, no. 3 (17 July 1980): 130–35.

5. Kenneth Manton, "Changing Concepts of Morbidity and Mortality in the Elderly Population," *Milbank Memorial Fund Quarterly/Health and Society* 60, no. 2 (Spring 1982): 183–245.

References

ABBREVIATIONS USED IN TEXT REFERENCES

CBO	U.S. Congress. Congressional Budget Office.
Census	U.S. Department of Commerce. Bureau of the Census.
DHEW	U.S. Department of Health, Education, and Welfare.
GAO	U.S. General Accounting Office.
HCFA	U.S. Department of Health and Human Services. Health Care Financing Administration.
NCHS	U.S. Department of Health and Human Services. National Center for Health Statistics.
NCHSR	U.S. Department of Health and Human Services. National Center for Health Services Research.
OFAA	U.S. Department of Health and Human Services. Health Care Financing Administration. Office of Financial and Actuarial Analysis.
OMB	U.S. Office of Management and Budget.
Senate	U.S. Congress. Senate.

Aday, LuAnn, Ronald Anderson, and Gretchen Fleming. 1980. *Health Care in the U.S.: Equitable for Whom?* Beverly Hills: Sage Publications.

Alpha Center. 1984. "Long Term Care Alternatives: Continuing Care Retirement Communities." *Alpha Centerpiece* (Bethesda, Md.) (January), pp. 1–6.

Anderson, Gerard, and James Knickman. 1984. "Patterns of Expenditures Among High Utilizers of Medical Care Services." *Medical Care* (February), pp. 143–49.

Auerbach, Arnold J. 1982. "Medicare Plan C: A Long Term Care Proposal." *Generations* 7 (Spring): 48–53.

Berg, Robert L., Francis E. Browning, John G. Hill, and Walter Wenkert. 1970. "Assessing the Health Care Needs of the Aged." *Health Services Research* (Spring): 36–59.

Berk A., L. C. Pannger, and T. D. Woolsey. 1978. "Estimating Deaths for the United States in 1900 by Cause, Age, and Sex." *Public Health Reports* 93, no. 5 (September-October): 479–82.

Bishop, Christine E. 1980. "A Compulsory National Long Term Care Insurance Program." In *Reforming the Long Term Care System*, edited by James J. Callahan, Jr. and Stanley S. Wallack, 61–94. Lexington, Mass.: Lexington Books.

Bjornstad, Penny. 1984. "Tax Benefits for Long-term Care of the Elderly: The Idaho Experience." Presentation at Conference on Long-Term Care Financing and Delivery Systems: Exploring Some Alternatives, sponsored by HCFA, Washington, D.C., 24 January.

Butler, Lewis, and Paul Newacheck. 1982. "Sociodemographic Characteristics of the Aged." In *Policy Options in Long Term Care*, edited by Judith Meltzer, Frank Farrow, and Harold Richmond, 38–77. Chicago: University of Chicago Press.

Butler, Robert. 1975. *Why Survive: Being Old in America*. New York: Harper and Row.

Callahan, James, Larry Diamond, J. Giele, and R. Morris. 1980. "Responsibilities of Families for Their Severely Disabled Elderly." *Health Care Financing Review* 1, no. 3 (Winter): 29–49.

Cohen, Joel. 1983. "Public Programs Financing Long Term Care." Urban Institute Working Paper no. 1466-18. Washington, D.C.: Urban Institute. January.

Davis, Carolyne. 1983. Testimony. Hearing on the future of Medicare. U.S. Congress, Senate, Special Committee on Aging. Washington, D.C., 13 April.

Davis, Karen. 1983. "Health Implications of Aging in America." Presentation at conference on the Impact of Technology on Aging in America, sponsored by the U.S. Congress, Office of Technology Assessment, Millwood, Va., 16–18 February.

Davis, Karen, and Diane Rowland. 1984. "Medicare Financing Reform: A New Medicare Premium." In U.S. Congress, House, Committee on Ways and Means, Subcommittee on Health, *Proceedings of the Conference on the Future of Medicare.* Washington, D.C.: U.S. Government Printing Office.

Diamond, Larry M., and David E. Berman. 1980. "The Social Health Maintenance Organization: A Single Entry, Prepaid, Long-Term-Care Delivery System." In *Reforming the Long Term Care System*, edited by James J. Callahan, Jr. and Stanley S. Wallack, 185–213. Lexington, Mass.: Lexington Books.

Dobson, Allen, Jack Scharff, and Larry Corder. 1983. "Six Months of Medicaid Data: A Summary from the National Medical Care Utilization and Expenditure Survey." *Health Care Financing Review* 4, no. 3 (March): 115–21.

Donabedian, Avedis. 1976. "Effects of Medicare and Medicaid on Access to and Quality of Health Care." *Public Health Reports* 91, no. 4 (July–August): 322–31.

Drake, David F. 1978. "Does Money Spent on Health Care Really Improve U.S. Health Status?" *Hospitals* 52 (16 October): 63–65.

Etheredge, Lynn. 1983. Testimony. U.S. Congress, House, Committee on Energy and Commerce, Subcommittee on Health and the Environment. 18 July.

Farrow, Frank, Tom Joe, Judith Meltzer, and Harold Richmond. 1982. "The Framework and Directions for Change." In *Policy Options in Long Term Care*, edited by Judith Meltzer, Frank Farrow, and Harold Richmond, 1–37. Chicago: University of Chicago Press.

Feder, Judith, and William Scanlon. 1982. "The Underused Benefit: Medicare's Coverage of Nursing Home Care." *Milbank Memorial Fund Quarterly/Health and Society* 60, no. 4 (Fall): 604–32.

Ferry, T. P., M. Gornick, M. Newton, and C. Hacherman. 1980. "Physicians' Charges Under Medicare: Assignment Rates and Beneficiary Liability." *Health Care Financing Review* 1, no. 3 (Winter): 49–73.

Firman, James. 1983. "Reforming Community Care for the Elderly and Disabled." *Health Affairs* (Millwood, Va.: Project Hope) 2, no. 1 (Spring): 66–82.

Fisher, Charles R. 1980. "Differences by Age Groups in Health Care Spending." *Health Care Financing Review* 1, no. 4 (Spring): 65–90.

Fox, Peter D. 1984. "Physician Reimbursement Under Medicare: An Overview and a Proposal for Areawide Physician Incentives." In U.S. Congress, House, Committee on Ways and Means, Subcommittee on Health, *Proceedings of the Conference on the Future of Medicare.* Washington, D.C.: U.S. Government Printing Office.

Fox, Peter D., and Stephen B. Clauser. 1980. "Trends in Nursing Home Expenditures: Implications for Aging Policy." *Health Care Financing Review* 2, no. 2 (Fall): 65–70.

Freeland, Mark, and Carol Schendler. 1983. "National Health Expenditures Growth in the 1980's: An Aging Population, New Technologies, and Increasing Competition." *Health Care Financing Review* 4, no. 3 (March): 1–59.

Friedman, B. 1976. "Mortality, Disability, and the Normative Economics of Medicare." In *The Role of Health Insurance in the Health Services Sector*, edited by Richard N. Rossett, 365–90. New York: National Bureau of Economic Research.

Fries, James F. 1980. "Aging, Natural Death, and the Compression of Morbidity." *New England Journal of Medicine* 303, no. 3 (17 July): 130–35.

Fullerton, William D. 1982. "Finding the Money and Paying for Long Term Care Services: The Devil's Briarpatch." In *Policy Options in Long Term Care*, edited by Judith Meltzer, Frank Farrow, and Harold Richmond, 182–208. Chicago: University of Chicago Press.

———. 1984. "Favorable Tax Treatment for the Elderly." Presentation at Conference on Long-Term Care Financing and Delivery Systems: Exploring Some Alternatives, sponsored by HCFA, Washington, D.C., 24 January.

Gibson, Robert M., Daniel R. Waldo, and Katharine R. Levit. 1983. "National Health Expenditures, 1982." *Health Care Financing Review* 5, no. 1 (Fall): 1–31.

Ginsburg, Paul B., and Marilyn Moon. 1984. "An Introduction to the Medicare Financing Problem." In U.S. Congress, House, Committee on Ways and Means, Subcommittee on Health, *Proceedings of the Conference on the Future of Medicare.* Washington, D.C.: U.S. Government Printing Office.

Gornick, Marion, James Beebe, and Ronald Prihoda. 1983. "Options for Change Under Medicare: Impact of a Cap on Catastrophic Illness Expense." *Health Care Financing Review* 5, no. 1 (Fall): 33–43.

Greenberg, Jay, and Walter N. Leutz. 1984. "The Social/Health Maintenance

Organization and its Role in Reforming the Long-term Care System." Presentation at Conference on Long-Term Care Financing and Delivery Systems: Exploring Some Alternatives, sponsored by HCFA, Washington, D.C., 24 January.

Gruenberg, Ernest M. 1977. "The Failures of Success." *Milbank Memorial Fund Quarterly/Health and Society* 55 (Winter): 3–24.

Gruenberg, Leonard W., and Karl A. Pillemer. 1980. "Disability Allowance for Long Term Care." In *Reforming the Long Term Care System*, edited by James J. Callahan, Jr. and Stanley S. Wallack, 95–117. Lexington, Mass.: Lexington Books.

Helbing, Charles. 1983. "Medicare: Use and Reimbursement for Aged Persons by Survival Status, 1979." Health Care Financing Notes, no. 1, November. Publication no. HCFA 03166. Baltimore.

Hsiao, William, and Nancy L. Kelly. 1984. "Restructuring Medicare Benefits." In U.S. Congress, House, Committee on Ways and Means, Subcommittee on Health, *Proceedings of the Conference on the Future of Medicare.* Washington, D.C.: U.S. Government Printing Office.

Hudson, Robert B. 1980. "Restructuring Federal/State Relations in Long Term Care: The Block Grant Alternative." In *Reforming the Long Term Care System,* edited by James J. Callahan, Jr. and Stanley S. Wallack, 31–59. Lexington, Mass.: Lexington Books.

———. 1981. "A Block Grant to the States for Long Term Care." *Journal of Health Politics, Policy, and Law* 6, no. 1 (Spring): 9–28.

Jacobs, Bruce, and William Weissert. 1984. "Home Equity Financing of Long-term Care for the Elderly." Presentation at Conference on Long-Term Care Financing and Delivery Systems: Exploring Some Alternatives, sponsored by HCFA, Washington, D.C., 24 January.

Keeler, Emmett B., David H. Solomon, John C. Beck, Robert C. Mendenhall, and Robert L. Kane. 1982. "Effect of Patient Age in Duration of Medical Encounters with Physicians." *Medical Care* 20, no. 11 (November): 1101–8.

Klarman, Herbert E. 1967. "Present Status of Cost-Benefit Analysis in the Health Field." *American Journal of Public Health* 57 (November): 1948–53.

———. 1982. "The Road to Cost-Effectiveness Analysis." *Milbank Memorial Fund Quarterly/Health and Society* 60, no. 4 (Fall): 585–603.

Kleinman, Joel C., Marsha Gold, and Diane Makuc. 1981. "Use of Ambulatory Medical Care by the Poor: Another Look at Equity." *Medical Care* 19, no. 10 (October): 1011–29.

Kovar, Mary Grace. 1982. "Health of the U.S. Elderly." Presentation at American Public Health Association Annual Meeting, Montreal, November.

———. 1983. "The United States Elderly People and Their Medical Care." Background paper for Commonwealth Fund Forum 1983 on Improving the Health of the Homebound Elderly, London, May.

Kramer, Morton. 1980. "The Rising Pandemic of Mental Disorders and Associated Chronic Diseases and Disabilities." In "Epidemiological Research as a Basis for the Organization of Extramural Psychiatry," *Acta Psychiatrica Scandinavia,* Supplement 285, 62: 382–96.

Kutza, Elizabeth. 1981. *The Benefits of Old Age.* Chicago: University of Chicago Press.

Lave, Judith R. 1984. "Hospital Payment under Medicare." In U.S. Congress, House, Committee on Ways and Means, Subcommittee on Health, *Proceedings of the Conference on the Future of Medicare.* Washington, D.C.: U.S. Government Printing Office.

Lifson, Arthur. 1984. "Long-term Care: An Insurer's Perspective." Presentation at Conference on Long-Term Care Financing and Delivery Systems: Exploring Some Alternatives, sponsored by HCFA, Washington, D.C., 24 January.

Link, Charles R., Stephen H. Long, and Russell F. Settle. 1980. "Costsharing, Supplementary Insurance, and Health Services Utilization Among the Medicare Elderly." *Health Care Financing Review* 2, no. 2 (Fall): 25–31.

Liu, Kenneth, Kenneth G. Manton, and Wiley S. Alliston. 1983. "Demographic and Epidemiologic Determinants of Expenditures." In *Long Term Care: Perspectives from Research and Demonstrations,* edited by Ronald J. Vogel and Hans C. Palmer, 81–102. Baltimore: HCFA.

Long, Stephen, and Thomas Smeeding. 1984. "Alternative Financing Sources." In U.S. Congress, House, Committee on Ways and Means, Subcommittee on Health, *Proceedings of the Conference on the Future of Medicare.* Washington, D.C.: U.S. Government Printing Office.

Lowenstein, Regina. 1971. "The Effects of Medicare on the Health Care of the Aged." *Social Security Bulletin* 34, no. 4 (April): 3–30.

Lowy, Lewis. 1981. *Social Policies for the Aged.* Cambridge, Mass.: Lexington Books.

Lubitz, James, and Ronald Deacon. 1982. "The Rise in Incidence of Hospitalizations Among the Aged, 1967 to 1979." *Health Care Financing Review* 3, no. 3 (March): 21–40.

Lubitz, James, Marion Gornick, and Ron Prihoda. 1981. "Use and Cost of Medicare Services in the Last Year of Life." HCFA Working Paper. Baltimore. 21 September.

McCall, N., and H. S. Wai. 1983. "An Analysis of the Use of Medicare Services by the Continuously Enrolled Aged." *Medical Care* 6 (June 21): 567–85.

McMillan, Alma, Penelope Pine, Marion Gornick, and Ronald Prihoda. 1983. "A Study of the Cross-over Population: Aged Persons Entitled to Both Medicare and Medicaid." *Health Care Financing Review* 4, no. 4 (Summer): 19–46.

Manton, Kenneth. 1982. "Changing Concepts of Morbidity and Mortality in the Elderly Population." *Milbank Memorial Fund Quarterly/Health and Society* 60, no. 2 (Spring): 183–245.

Medicare Board of Trustees. 1983. "Summary of the 1983 Annual Reports of the Medicare Board of Trustees." *Health Care Financing Review* 5, no. 2 (Winter): 1–10.

Meiners, Mark. 1983a. "The Case for Long Term Care Insurance." *Health Affairs* 2, no. 2 (Summer): 55–79.

———. 1983b. "The State of the Art in Long Term Care Insurance." NCHSR Working Paper. July.

Meiners, Mark, and Gordon R. Trapnell. 1984. "Long Term Care Insurance:

Premium Estimates for Prototype Policies." *Medical Care* 22, no. 10 (October): 901–11.

Merriam, I. A. 1964. Testimony. Hearing on Blue Cross and other private health insurance for the elderly. U.S. Congress, Senate, Special Committee on Aging. Subcommittee on Health of the Elderly, Document no. 88:2, pt. 1, pp. 3–13. Washington, D.C.: U.S. Government Printing Office.

Mossey, J. M., and E. Shapiro. 1982. "Self-rated Health: A Predictor of Mortality Among the Elderly." *American Journal of Public Health* 72, no. 8 (August): 800–808.

Muse, Donald. 1982. *National Annual Medicaid Statistics: Fiscal Years 1973–1979.* Baltimore: HCFA.

Nagi, Saad Z. 1976. "Epidemiology of Disability among Adults in the United States." *Milbank Memorial Fund Quarterly* 54, no. 4 (Fall): 439–69.

National Study Group on State Medicaid Strategies. 1984. "Restructuring Medicaid: An Agenda for Change." Available from the Center for the Study of Social Policy, 236 Massachusetts Ave., N.E., Washington, D.C. 20002.

Newhouse, Joseph, Willard G. Manning, Carl N. Morris, Carry L. Orr, Naihua Duan, Emmett B. Keeler, Arleen Leibowitz, Kent H. Marquis, M. Susan Marquis, Charles E. Phelphs, and Robert H. Brook. 1981. "Some Interim Results from a Controlled Trial of Cost-sharing in Health Insurance." *New England Journal of Medicine* 305, no. 25 (17 December): 1501–7.

Okun, Arthur M. 1975. *Equality and Efficiency: The Big Tradeoff.* Washington, D.C.: Brookings Institution.

Paringer, Lyn, James Bluck, Judy Feder, and John Holahan. 1979. *Health Status and Use of Medical Services.* Washington, D.C.: Urban Institute.

Pollack, William. 1983. "Financing Long Term Care: Promises and Principles." Presentation at conference on the Impact of Technology on Aging in America, sponsored by the U.S. Congress, Office of Technology Assessment, Millwood, Va., 16–18 February.

Rivlin, Alice. 1983. Testimony. Hearing on the future of Medicare. U.S. Congress, Senate, Special Committee on Aging. Washington, D.C., 13 April.

Roos, Noralou P., and Evelyn Shapiro. 1981. "The Manitoba Longitudinal Study on Aging: Preliminary Findings in Health Care Utilization by the Elderly." *Medical Care* 19, no. 6 (June): 644–57.

Rosenwaike, I., N. Yaffe, and P. C. Sagi. 1980. "The Recent Decline in Mortality of the Extreme Aged: An Analysis of Statistical Data." *American Journal of Public Health* 70, no. 10 (October): 1074–80.

Sangl, Judith A. 1983. "The Family Support System." In *Long Term Care: Perspectives from Research and Demonstrations,* edited by Ronald J. Vogel and Hans C. Palmer, 307–36. Baltimore: HCFA.

Scanlon, William J. 1980. "Toward a Theory of the Nursing Home Market." *Inquiry* 17 (Spring): 25–41.

Soldo, Beth J. 1980. "America's Elderly in the 1980's." *Population Bulletin* 35, no. 4 (November): 3–47.

Somers, Anne R. 1980. "Rethinking Health Policy for the Elderly: A 6-Point Program." *Inquiry* 17 (Spring): 3–17.

————. 1982. "Long Term Care for the Elderly and Disabled: A New Health Priority." *New England Journal of Medicine* 307, no. 4 (22 July): 221–26.

Storfer, Miles. 1981. "Medicaid Data Report July-September, 1980." Working Paper no. ER-MED-3-80. City of New York, Human Resources Administration. January.

Svanborg, Alvar. 1981. "Survey of Epidemiological Studies on Social and Medical Conditions of the Elderly." In *Workshop on Policy Oriented Research in the Health of the Elderly*, 20–21. Copenhagen: World Health Organization. July.

U.S. Congress. Congressional Budget Office. 1977. *Long Term Care for the Elderly and Disabled.* Washington, D.C.: U.S. Government Printing Office.

————. 1983. *Changing the Structure of Medicare Benefits: Issue and Options.* Washington, D.C.: Government Printing Office. March.

————. Senate. 1983. S. 1539. 98th Congress.

————. Senate. Special Committee on Aging. 1984. Staff estimates, personal communication.

U.S. Department of Commerce. Bureau of the Census. 1982. *Demographic Aspects of Aging and the Older Population in the United States.* Current Population Reports, series P-23, no. 59. Washington, D.C.: U.S. Government Printing Office.

————. 1983. *America in Transition: An Aging Society.* Current Population Reports, Special Studies, series P-23, no. 128. Washington, D.C.: U.S. Government Printing Office, September.

U.S. Department of Health and Human Services. Health Care Financing Administration. 1981. *Long Term Care: Background and Future Directions.* Publication no. HCFA 81-20047. Washington, D.C. January.

————. 1982. *Medicare and Medicaid Data Book, 1981.* Publication no. HCFA 03128. Baltimore.

————. 1983a. *Medicare and Medicaid Data Book, 1983.* Publication no. HCFA 03156. Baltimore. December.

————. 1983b. *Annual Medicare Program Statistics, 1981.* Publication no. HCFA 03153. Baltimore.

————. 1983c. "HCFA Program Statistics." *Health Care Financing Review* 4, no. 3 (March): 127–32.

————. 1983d. "Health Care Financing Trends." *Health Care Financing Review* 5, no. 1 (Fall): 103–5.

U.S. Department of Health and Human Services. Health Care Financing Administration. Office of Financial and Actuarial Analysis. 1982. Unpublished statistics. Baltimore.

U.S. Department of Health and Human Services. National Center for Health Statistics. 1981. *Characteristics of Nursing Home Residents, Health Status, and Care Received: National Nursing Home Survey, United States, May-December 1977.* DHHS Publication no. (PHS) 81-1712. Washington, D.C.: U.S. Government Printing Office.

————. 1982. *Health, United States, 1981,* DHHS Publication no. (PHS) 82-1232, Washington, D.C.: U.S. Government Printing Office.

————. 1983a. *Health, United States, 1982.* DHHS Publication no. (PHS) 83-1232. Washington, D.C.: U.S. Government Printing Office.

————. 1983b. Unpublished statistics from 1980 National Medical Care Expenditure and Utilization Survey.

U.S. Department of Health and Human Services. National Center for Health Services Research. 1982. "National Medical Care Expenditure Survey, 1977." Unpublished statistics. Hyattsville, Md.

U.S. Department of Health, Education, and Welfare. 1978. *Health: United States, 1976–1977.* DHEW Publication no. (PHS) 77-1232. Washington, D.C.: U.S. Government Printing Office.

————. 1980. *Health, United States, 1979.* DHEW Publication no. (PHS) 80-1232. Washington, D.C.: U.S. Government Printing Office.

U.S. General Accounting Office. 1979. *Entering a Nursing Home: Costly Implications for Medicaid and the Elderly.* Washington, D.C.: U.S. Government Printing Office.

U.S. Office of Management and Budget. 1983. *Budget of the Government of the United States, FY 1984.* Washington, D.C.: U.S. Government Printing Office.

Vogel, Ronald J., and Hans Palmer. 1983. *Long Term Care: Perspectives from Research and Demonstrations,* Introduction. Baltimore: HCFA.

Weinrobe, Maurice. 1984. "Home Equity Conversion: Its Practice Today." Presentation at Conference on Long-Term Care Financing and Delivery Systems: Exploring Some Alternatives, sponsored by HCFA, Washington, D.C., 24 January.

Weissert, William. 1982. "Size and Characteristics of the Non-Institutionalized Long Term Care Population." Urban Institute Working Paper no. 1466-20. Washington, D.C.: Urban Institute. September.

Weissert, William, and William Scanlon. 1982. "Determinants of Institutionalization of the Aged." Urban Institute Working Paper no. 1466-21. Washington, D.C.: Urban Institute. September.

————. 1983. "Determinants of Institutionalization of the Aged." In *Final Report: Project to Analyze Existing Long Term Care Data,* vol. 3. DHHS Contract 100-80-0158, July.

Wilensky, Gail, and Mark Berk. 1983. "Medicare and the Elderly Poor." Hearing on the future of Medicare. U.S. Congress, Senate, Special Committee on Aging. Washington, D.C., 13 April.

Wilson, Peter A. 1981. "Hospital Use by the Aging Population." *Inquiry* 18, no. 4 (Winter): 332–44.

Winklevoss, Howard, and Alwyn V. Powell. 1984. *Continuing Care Retirement Communities: An Empirical, Financial, and Legal Analysis.* Pension Research Council of the Wharton School. Homewood, Ill.: Richard D. Irwin.

Index

Access: to long-term care, 114; Medicare and, 45; to nursing homes, 28; to services, 22

Acute care: integration of Medicare and Medicaid programs and, 111–20; Medicaid and, 106; Medicare and, 27, 69; utilization of services and, 27

Administration: integration of Medicaid and Medicare programs and, 120; organization of services and, 2–3

Aid to Families with Dependent Children (AFDC), 55

Age: characteristics of elderly and, 7, 9, 11; hospital utilization and, 22, 25; nursing home utilization and, 28, 29

Alcohol tax, 84

Alliston, Wiley S., 20

Ambulatory care, 33, 82

American Medical Association, 82

Arteriosclerosis, 28

Arthroplasty, 26

Assessment: preadmission, 113; self-assessment of health, 11, 16

Benefits, 2, 56–60, 111

Blacks. See Race

Block grants, 100–104

Canada, 13, 16, 26, 27, 30, 124

CAP. See Computer Assisted Planning model of health system

Cardiac surgery, 25

Care, channeling of, 71, 94

Case management, 70, 94

Cash grants, 104–5

Cataract operations, 26

Chronic conditions, 11, 16–20, 24, 28, 41, 68

Cigarette tax, 84, 115

Community-based service grants, 103–4

Computer Assisted Planning (CAP) model of health system, 123–24

Consumer reform incentives, 74–79, 87–94. See also Reform

Coronary bypass, 26

Cost controls, 120

Cost sharing, 75–77, 108

Data: CAP model and, 123; demographic, 1, 7–11; health status, 11–22

Delivery system reform, 94–100. See also Reform

Demographic data: of elderly, 7–11; projected elderly, 1. See also Data

Demonstration projects, 70–71, 94, 113

Department of Health and Human Services, 29, 71, 123

Department of Housing and Urban Development, 68

Dependence, 11, 20–21, 28

Diagnosis related groups (DRGs), 79–81

Disability, 103, 124; health status analysis and, 7, 11, 16–20; long-term care insurance and, 106; nursing homes and, 18; physical impairment, 68; prevalence in very old, 7

Disability allowances, 104–5

Discharges, 24, 80

Divorce, 21

Drake, David F., 45

Elderly: demographic characteristics of,
   7–11; financing sources of, 33–34;
   health expenditures as burden of, 34–
   36; health needs and financial resource conflict of, 1–2; health status
   of, 11–22; importance of Medicad to
   poor, 48; importance of Medicare to
   poor, 3–4; income of, 35; integration
   of Medicaid and Medicare programs
   and, 114; reform in health care for,
   2–3
Eligibility: gaps in, 69; Medicaid, 51–56,
   61, 100, 101, 102; welfare and Medicaid, 50
Emergency room, 23, 30
Entitlement programs (grants), 100–104
Entry evaluation, 70
Etheredge, Lynn, 82
Expenditures. See Health care expenditures

Families: composition of, 9–10; dependence and, 20–21; long-term care and,
   62, 89; support of, 11, 62, 89, 104,
   113
Federal government: health needs and financial resource conflict and, 1–2;
   long-term care and, 62. See also Medicaid; Medicare
Financial resources: health care for elderly and, 3; integration of Medicaid
   and Medicare programs and, 111–12;
   long-term care reforms and, 71–73
Forecasting, CAP model and, 123–24
Fox, Peter D., 82
Friedman, B., 45
Fries, James F., 13

Gephardt, Congressman, 77
Government. See Federal government;
   State government
Gradison, Congressman, 77
Grants (block), 100–104
Gruenberg, Ernest M., 20, 124

Health care expenditures: acute care
   and, 27; deficits of HI Trust Fund
   and, 46–48; DRGs and, 79–81; dying
   patients and Medicare, 43; for elderly,

3; families and nursing home, 62, 89;
   as financial burden for elderly, 34–36;
   financing sources for elderly and, 33–
   34; home health care, 66; increase in
   Medicare, 36–37; long-term care, 62–
   63, 86; Medicaid trends in, 51, 60;
   Medicaid type, 56; Medicare trends in,
   39–44; rising costs of SMI and, 47–
   48; survey of, 29, 76
Health care industry, 1–2
Health insurance. See Insurance
Health maintenance organizations
   (HMOs), 78; social (S/HMO), 95–97,
   99
Health status: chronic conditions, 11,
   16–20; dependence and, 11, 20–21;
   disability and, 7, 11, 16–20; hospital
   use and, 24; income and, 20–21; life
   expectancy and, 11, 12–16; Medicare
   and, 45; morbidity and, 11; mortality
   rates and, 11, 12–16, 45; physician
   use and, 23; race and, 20–21; residence and, 21; self-assessment of, 11,
   16
Health system model, 123–24
Home care, 28; Medicaid and, 65; Medicare and, 63, 65–66; volunteers for,
   113
Home-equity conversion concept, 87–89
Hospital Insurance (HI), 38–39, 66, 110
Hospital Insurance (HI) Trust Fund,
   114; deficits, 46–48, 72; Medicare
   premiums and, 84, 85; payroll tax
   and, 83–84
Hospitals, 111; delivery system reform
   and, 94–100; Medicare payment practices and, 37; Medicare reform and,
   79–81; teaching, 79
Hospital services utilization, 23–27, 41,
   45, 58, 117; cost sharing and, 75–77

Idaho, 94
Income: of elderly, 35; health status and,
   20–21; long-term care and, 88; services and, 26, 30
Income-related premium, 115–16
Insurance: coinsurance and, 74, 75–77,
   116; elderly and, 35–36; employment,
   32; HI, 38–39, 46–48, 66, 72, 83–

84, 85, 110, 111, 114; hospitalizations and, 25–26; Medicare coverage available, 38–39; Medicare expansion and public, 107–9; private, 36, 77–79, 89–92; public, 105–7; SMI, 35–36, 38–39, 46, 47–48, 50, 66, 78, 81, 82, 84–85, 89, 95, 109, 110, 111–12

Intermediate care facility (ICF), 56, 63

Johns Hopkins University, 123

Kovar, Mary Grace, 16
Kramer, Morton, 20, 124

Length of stay, Medicare reform and, 76
Life care communities, 97–100
Life expectancy, 11, 12–16
Liu, Kenneth, 20
Longevity, 45
Long-term care: access to, 114; block grants through states and, 100–104; consumer incentives for reform and, 87–94; defining, 62; delivery system and reform of, 94–100; demonstration projects and, 70–71; disability allowances and, 104–5; families and, 62, 89; federal deficits and, 1; financial reforms and, 71–73; integration of Medicaid and Medicare and, 111–20; Medicare expansion and, 107–9; problems with, 68–70; public expenditures for, 62–63; public insurance and, 105–7; public programs for, 63–68; utilization of services and, 27–29

Maine, 60
Manton, Kenneth, 13, 20, 124
Marital patterns, 10
Medicaid: accomplishments of, 60–61; acute care and, 106; benefits and, 56–60; cutbacks in, 1; demonstration projects and, 70, 94, 113; eligibility and, 51–56, 61, 100, 101, 102; expenditure survey and, 76; expenditure trends and, 51; financing and, 63; gaps in program of, 61; health expenditures and, 33–34, 35; home care and, 65; importance of (to elderly poor), 3–4; integration with Medicare and,

111–20; nursing homes and, 55–56, 58, 65, 69, 90; private insurance and, 91; public insurance and, 106; reform and, 71; service grants and, 103; as supplement to Medicare, 48–51, 60–61
Medicare, 4; accomplishments of, 44–45; acute care and, 27, 69; consumer incentives for reform and, 74–79; controversy and difficulties of, 36–37, 46; coverage available under, 38–39; cutbacks in, 1; demonstration projects and, 70, 94, 113; dying patients and, 43; expenditure increase and, 36–37; expenditure trends of, 39–44; financing and, 63; health expenditures and, 33–34, 35; HI and, 38–39, 46–48, 66, 72, 83–84, 85, 110, 111, 114; home care and, 63, 65–66; integration with Medicaid and, 111–20; Medicaid as supplement to, 48–51, 60–61; provider incentives for reform and, 79–83; public insurance and, 107–9; reform and, 71; revenue increases and reform and, 83–85; SMI and, 35–36, 38–39, 46, 47–48, 50, 66, 78, 81, 82, 84–85, 89, 95, 110, 111–12; use differentials and, 29
Medicare vouchers, 77–79
Medication, 56, 61
"Medigap" policies. See Medicare
Minorities, 30. See also Race
Morbidity, 11
Mortality rates, 11, 12–16, 45, 124

National Long-Term Care Channeling Project, 71, 94
National Medical Care Expenditure Survey, 29, 76
National Study Group on State Medicaid Strategies, 101
New Hampshire, 60
North Dakota, 60
Norway, 124
Nursing homes; age and sex and, 28, 29; dependence and, 20; disabilities and, 18; expenditures on, 32–33; financing and, 62, 63; Medicaid and, 55–56, 58, 65, 69, 90; private insurance and,

89–92; problem of supply of, 69; utilization of services of, 28–29

Older Americans Act, 68, 100, 103
Organizational effectiveness, 61, 62
Organizational restructuring, 94
Outpatient departments, 23, 30

Patient care. *See* Acute care; Home care; Long-term care
Payment. *See* Reimbursement
Payroll tax, 47, 83–84
Physical impairment, 68
Physicians, 111; Medicare reform and, 81–83; payments to, 114; SMI and, 39, 81, 82; utilization of services of, 22–23, 41; visits to, 22–23, 24, 60
Policy. *See* Public policy
Population: prediction of elderly, 1; present elderly, 7–11
Poverty, 20–21; Medicaid and, 48
Prepaid health plans, 77–79
Prescription drugs, 56, 61
Public policy; health sector, 1; reform in health care for elderly and, 2–3; social, 100

Quality care, 2

Race: health status and, 20–21; services and, 26, 29–30
Rand Corporation, 76
Reagan administration, 75, 81, 101
Reform: block grants through states and, 100–104; consumer incentives and, 74–79, 87–94; delivery system and, 94–100; developing and implementing long-term care, 86–87; disability allowances and, 104–5; in health care for elderly, 2–3; long-term care and financial, 71–73; provider incentives for, 79–83; public insurance and, 105–9; revenue increases and, 83–85
Reimbursement: cost sharing and, 75; DRGs and hospital, 79–81; hospitals and Medicare, 37; physician, 114; prepaid plans and, 77–79; prospective payment and, 113; provider, 112–13

Research, 70–71
Residence, 21, 26
Respite care, 113
Revenue increases (Medicare), 83–85
Rosenwaike, I., 45
Rural sector, 21

Savings accounts (personal), 92–93
Services: community-based grants and, 103–4; integration of Medicaid and Medicare programs and, 113; long-term care reform and, 94–100; organization of, 2–3; question of limits on, 2; utilization of acute care, 27; utilization of hospital, 23–27; utilization of long-term care, 27–39; utilization of physician, 22–23
Sex: chracteristics of elderly and, 7, 9, 11; hospital utilization and, 22; life expectancy and, 12; nursing home use and, 28, 29
Skilled nursing facility (SNF), 56, 63, 66
Social/health maintenance organization (S/HMO). *See* Health maintenance organizations
SMI (Supplementary Medical Insurance). *See* Medicare
State government: block grants and, 100–104; long-term care and, 62; Medicaid assistance and, 48, 50, 60
Supplemental Security Income, 50, 53, 56, 63, 67–68, 104
Support: dependence and family, 20–21; of families, 11, 62, 89, 104, 113
Surgery, 25, 26

Taxes, 117; alcohol and cigarette, 84, 115; consumer incentives for reform and, 92–94; general, 84; payroll, 47, 83–84
Tax surcharge, 115, 116
Technology, 124
TEFRA, 47
Texas, 60
Title XX program, 63, 67, 100, 103, 108

United Kingdom, 26

Vascular surgery, 25
Veterans Administration, 63, 67
Visits to physicians, 22–23, 24, 60. *See also* Physicians
Volunteers (home care), 113

Vouchers: cash, 104–5; Medicare, 77–79

Welfare, Medicaid eligibility and, 50
Wyoming, 60

Karen Davis, Ph.D., is professor and chairman of the Department of Health Policy and Management at the Johns Hopkins University School of Hygiene and Public Health. She has taught economics at Rice University and Harvard University and has been a research associate during several years at the Brookings Institution. She served in the Department of Health and Human Services from 1977 to 1981, where she was appointed Administrator of the Health Resources Administration of the U.S. Public Health Service. She is author or coauthor of *National Health Insurance: Benefits, Costs, and Consequences* and *Health and the War on Poverty: A Ten-Year Appraisal* and of two Social Security Administration monographs.

Diane Rowland, M.P.A., is working toward a doctorate in the Department of Health Policy and Management at Johns Hopkins, where she has been a research associate since 1981. She served as deputy to Karen Davis at the Department of Health and Human Services and succeeded her as acting Deputy Assistant Secretary for Planning and Evaluation. She has been a consultant at the Center for Health Policy Studies of the Georgetown University Medical Center.

The Johns Hopkins University Press

Medicare Policy

This book was composed in Goudy Old Style text and display type by EPS Group, Inc., from a design by Chris L. Smith. It was printed on 50-lb. S. D. Warren's Sebago Eggshell Cream Offset paper and bound in Holliston's Payko by the Maple Press Company.

DATE DUE

APR 2 9 1990			
NOV 1 3 1990			